RESTORING HEALTH:
Body, Mind and Spirit

FROM THE BOOK SERIES:
Strengthening a New Generation of Healthy Leaders

by The Reverend Dr. Ed Hird

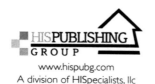

HISPUBLISHING
GROUP

www.hispubg.com
A division of HISpecialists, llc

Dr. Hird is a man of many talents. His writings are fun to read and are packed with knowledge that can be applied to our spiritual lives. I am very honoured to know him and to have read his books. There are two things that can change your life, the people you meet and the books you read. This book will change your life for the better.

Dr. Peter Eppinga M.D.
drpetereppinga.com

In *Restoring Health: Body, Mind and Spirit,* the Reverend Dr. Ed Hird takes us on an epic journey through the biblical book of Titus, Paul's instruction manual for the pirates on the island of Crete. Ed Hird develops the idea that we are all pirates, in need of salvation and holistic health in body, mind and spirit—in need of health in every area of our lives. He reminds us that Healthiness = Godliness = Christlikeness.

In the church today there is a desperate need for holistically healthy leaders—just as Titus the Greek Christian was to the Cretan pirates. The question remains—will we be available and accountable to God in choosing the way of health, of life and of godliness? I highly recommend this book to all who desire to choose the healthy way of Christlikeness.

John Cline MD, BSc, IFMCP
-author of the book *Detoxify for Life* | detoxifyforlife.com
Medical Director of the Cline Medical Centre in Nanaimo,
a licensed medical doctor in BC and certified by the
International Board of Clinical Metal Toxicology. He
is also medical director of the Oceanside Functional
Medicine Research Institute.

Dr. Hird has done it again. He has woven a thoroughly modern work in and through the Ancient Biblical text. His insights on the modern life are powerful and his discoveries in the ancient text are fascinating. Kudos to you Dr. Hird. We appreciate your powerful pen.

Dr. Gil Stieglitz
www.gilstieglitz.com
author of *Deep Happiness: The eight secrets* – a
powerful work exploring how to inject the
Beatitudes into our life.

A very engaging book. I especially have enjoyed the anecdotal stories that fortify your positions, not to mention the history lessons. I am becoming educated while becoming inspired.

Dr. Kevin Orieux
President, Aararat Consulting | www.aararat.com
Author of *Survive, Thrive or Dive* and *What's Your ROI?*

You have never read a Bible commentary like this. Paul's Letter to Titus could well be subtitled 'Pirates of the Mediterranean'. Dr Hird's highly readable style lights up Paul's counsel to his young friend whom he charges with discipling and training Piracy Island in the revolutionary courage of the truth of Jesus. This pastoral epistle sparkles with contemporary insight."

The Rev. Canon Dr. Chris Sugden
Trustee, *Anglican Mainstream*
www.anglican-mainstream.net

In this highly toxic world, we desperately need a 360-degrees restoration of our whole being, marriage, family, church, society and beyond. Dr. Hird gives us a Biblical and practical way to learn how Paul raised Titus so that we can let that restoration happen to us. A new generation of healthy leaders will be raised up because of our faithfulness and willingness.

The Right Rev. Dr. Silas Ng
Missionary Bishop, Anglican Mission in the Americas
www.theamia.org | www.theamcanada.ca

Couch potatoes beware! Ed Hird has written a book that both comforts the afflicted and afflicts the comfortable. *Restoring Health* is not just an energy bar. It is a spiritual blood transfusion. Hard-hitting, and yet grace-filled, this book will awaken you to 100 areas of your spiritual life that need reinvigorating. If you are a pastor, you will find innumerable nuggets of truth and a treasure store of illustrative material. Plus you will see how simple biblical exposition is—get the text right, and then illuminate it with a good illustration. If you are a lay person, watch out. Ed Hird will light a fire under you and challenge you to explosive discipleship.

Dr. Peter C. Moore
Dean/President Emeritus, Trinity School for Ministry, PA
and Associate for Discipleship, St. Michael's Church, Charleston, SC

petercmoore.com

Ed Hird opens up the book of Titus in a rich and provocative way that will help you become a better leader and follower of Jesus.

–Margaret Feinberg
author of *Wonderstruck*
www.margaretfeinberg.com

With immense gusto and zest, I would endorse the important content of your marvelous book that reflects the theology of human "Body Mind and Spirit."

Msgr. Pedro Lopez-Gallo
Pastor of St. Pius Church, North Vancouver (retired)

Full of personal and historical stories that illustrate the points he is making (which will not surprise anyone who knows Ed), the book reflects on the nature of Christian character and leadership, each meditation tied to a verse or half-verse of Titus with frequent reference to his overall theme of pirates turned into at least good people of faith, if not saints.

Peter H. Davids, Ph.D.
Visiting Professor of Theology, Houston Baptist University

What a joy and pleasure it is to read the completed commentary of Titus by the Rev. Dr. Ed Hird. I am so thankful to God that He did not allow Ed to give up on the writing of this commentary. Otherwise, we would have been deprived of this precious jewel which so richly, vividly and passionately reveals the inner heart of God. God raised up Christian leaders in every generation to confront the pirate character buried in every human heart.

Paul, recognizing the grace and peace of God in Titus, made a bold, courageous, visionary and strategic choice by sending young Titus to Crete as a missionary. It is in this context that God spoke to the pirates in Crete. However, His message is relevant to all of us in every land and in every generation. Modern-day piracy has effectively planted itself into the system of our churches. The pirating nature drains God's resources endowed to the churches for purpose of mission. It carries out its desire to deceive, rob, and side-track us from the Gospel of Jesus Christ. It sows false gospels into our lives. Ultimately, it destroys the church.

Ed's passion is now very much focused on the call to minister to the lives within the Canadian Anglican Church in North America. I am so grateful to God for the miracle of the completion of this book. My reading of this small commentary with a huge gospel truth has deeply impacted me and encouraged me to continue my journey to serve the Lord and to preach the Gospel. I highly recommend Dr. Ed Hird's book with a huge Gospel heart for the use of molding the leadership character of a new generation of healthy young leaders.

++Yong Ping Chung
Retired 2nd Primate of South East Asia and 4th Bishop of Sabah

Ed Hird's latest book on Titus, has unleashed a powerhouse of truth for the restoration of this generation. Through the apostle Paul's teaching accompanied by Ed's authentic and personal reflections, the reader is commanded to find truth and insights into how God has designed us to live and love.

Heidi McLaughlin
International Christian speaker & author of several books.
Member of AWSA, Word Guild. Wife, Step-mom, friend,
Golfer & Controller of VW Audi Dealership.
Kelowna, British Columbia.
heartconnection.ca

Ed Hird is a prophetic, courageous voice calling the church to be faithful to the whole gospel of Jesus Christ. *Restoring Health* draws its inspiration from Paul's letter to Titus and calls pastors and Christian leaders to become whole people—in mind, body, and spirit—who embody the whole gospel. Hird offers a powerful prescription for transforming of our lives and ministries into Spirit-filled witnesses to the Christ's power to restore not only our spirits, but our minds and bodies as well.

Ken Shigematsu
Senior pastor of Tenth Church, Vancouver,
and author of *God in My Everything*
Twitter.com/KenShigematsu
Facebook.com/GodInMyEverything

Ed's book, *Restoring Health: Body, Mind and Spirit*, brings fresh and captivating insights into Paul's letter to Titus. His explanation and analogy of pirates was brilliant. He is certainly on target in reaching and equipping the next generation.

David Koop, Coastal Church
Senior Pastor, Dr. (DMIN) | www.coastalchurch.org

Ed Hird has written a most engaging commentary on Titus, an easy read with informative insights into the lives of pirate Cretans and how we can learn from them today. If the good news of Jesus can impact that rebellious island, then Hird assures us that there is relevance and encouragement for our day. Pages are filled with interesting anecdotes and Hird's wide-ranging general knowledge makes for a thoroughly enjoyable read with many opportunities to pause and reflect along the way.

John Cox
Senior Pastor, Jericho Road | www.jerichoroad-church.com
author of *Googling God* | googleforgod.wordpress.com

Rev. Dr. Ed Hird, pastor and author, student of the Bible and human nature, has an ability to communicate and connect clearly through his writing. In his latest book *Restoring Health: Body, Mind and Spirit*, he relates Paul's letter to Titus to a comprehensive understanding of Cretian history and culture. He shares stories from his own and famous lives, and applies the lessons to a variety of real life practical and spiritual issues.

I love the way he explores the pirate culture, fact and fiction, and shows the"pirate" in all of us. Healthy living, in body, mind and spirit is a popular resolution today. The author shows God's way as to how this can be accomplished, not only in our personal lives, but in society as well.

The Rev. Dr Rod Ellis, Rector
Church of our Lord, Victoria | churchofourlord.org
Author of the book *King of Hearts*
www.amazon.com/King-Hearts-Rod-Ellis-ebook/dp/B00DU2XOW6

In *Restoring Health: Body, Mind and Spirit,* the Reverend Dr. Ed Hird offers readers a richly engaging devotional commentary on St. Paul's letter to Titus.

Each of Ed's chapters, in following the text of Paul's letter, skillfully interleaves well-informed exegesis with travelogue, history, personal and family autobiography, while also drawing on theological reflections from wise commentators—both ancient and modern, from Eusebius to Johnny Cash. Principal themes in Ed's study include teaching on how this Epistle can build up the spiritual, mental and physical health of Christians and church leaders, the importance of sound doctrine, and the vital operation of the gifts of the Holy Spirit—as necessary for today's Christians as for the Apostolic church.

In short, this clearly-written and very readable book offers valuable teaching on how the Gospel of Christ transformed the ancient Cretans and can do the same in our lives today. It also would serve as a superb resource for home and group Bible studies.

Dr. George Egerton
Professor Emeritus, UBC History Department
Editor, *Anglican Essentials*
ubcgcu.org/2012/10/19/george-egerton-professor-emeritus-history-ubc

Ed's writing ability engages you with the content and makes it real enough to want to live it. He's scholarly, practical and spiritual in a most wonderful way. Keep writing, Ed. Give us more.

Doug Schneider
Senior Pastor, The Embassy, Oshawa ON
theembassychurch.ca

This commentary on Titus is not just a devotional. It is a rallying cry for the Kingdom of God! It brings Titus out of relative obscurity into the front ranks of the 1st Century Apostles. We see Titus confronting the powers of darkness in ancient Crete with the Gospel and bringing transformation. A much needed message for anyone who loves their city and nation and feels in a rut.

Pastor David Carson
Vice Chair, Hope Vancouver

This book is so much more than a helpful resource for leaders. Rich in biblical insights, it offers any Christian the valuable tools needed to develop genuine character and a healthy spiritual life. Our generation is crying out for fathers who can help us grow--and Ed Hird is one of those fathers. I am honored to know him and to feed on the revelations he offers in this amazing book. This book sharpened my leadership skills and challenged me to pursue integrity, character and humility in my ministry. I know it will do the same for you.

J. Lee Grady
Former editor, *Charisma* magazine
Author, *The Holy Spirit Is Not for Sale*
Director, The Mordecai Project

Dr. Ed Hird+ has, once again, blessed the Christian Church with a clear, concise, contemporary, faithful, and pointed exposition of the Book of Titus. This book will be a source of spiritual health, liberation, restoration, and strength to Christian leaders, Christian homes, and God's world and anyone who cares to pick it up and read. I highly commend and recommend it to you and your church.

The Rt. Rev'd Dr. Felix Orji, OSB
Bishop: Anglican Diocese of the West(CANA/ACNA),
Church of Nigeria(Anglican Communion)
Anglican Cathedral Church of St. Francis, El Paso,Texas
stfrancisanglicanchurch.org

I highly recommend that you purchase Ed Hird's latest book *Restoring Health: Body, Mind and Spirit,* right away! Ed's insights come from his many fruitful years as a successful Pastor on the front lines of ministry in Canada. In addition, Ed is highly respected for his visionary leadership on a national level.

David Arrol Macfarlane
Director of National Initiatives
Billy Graham Evangelistic Association of Canada
www.billygraham.ca

Someone once stated "People buy into the leader long before they buy into his message." If this is the case, then please take a long look into my friend Ed Hird's latest book *Restoring Health: Body, Mind and Spirit.* Written out of the storehouse of his heart and ministry, Ed draws on the life of Titus ("an enthusiastic missional leader") in a way that compels us to live with integrity the call to healthy, Biblical, Kingdom leadership. A truly refreshing work!

Steve Schroeder
President, Christian Ministers Association of Canada
canadacma.org

This is one of the most fascinating books I have read in a long time and as a commentary rivals the work of Barclay. To expound the Biblical text, Ed brings in a wealth of contemporary examples that really bring it alive. Thus the book is a highly informative delight to read which I strongly recommend.

Dr. Irving Hexham, PhD,
Professor of Religious Studies,
University of Calgary and author of the website
www.understandingworldreligions.com

Ed Hird writes — "healthy leadership is about strengthening our spiritual sons and daughters in our common faith." — this captures the heart of his new book which will help us all strengthen a new generation of healthy leaders in the church as we learn from Paul's discipling of Titus.

The Reverend Canon William Beasley
Director of the Greenhouse Movement
www.greenhousemovement.com

Ed Hird is one of Canada's true treasures and humble Christian leaders. He is expertly qualified to guide the eager student through the New Testament epistle of Titus as it emphasizes the connection of doctrine—committed to faithful men—with holiness of life.

Tom Nisbett, Ph.D.
CFRE

Ed Hird's latest book is "unputtabledownable." *Restoring Health: Body, Mind and Spirit,* a study of Titus, is racy, deep, funny, wise, sober, radical, illustrative of to-day's dilemas and pertinent as to Christian answers to them. The fact he and his wife went to Crete, studied "the pirates" as he calls them, unveils and illustrates to us from the very locus the social, political, religious and historic settings out of which Titus is written grips and enlightens us on every page. Ed cleverly weaves Crete's real people of that time with today's people, the modern world, modern church, and in so doing unmasks our hypocrisies, our weaknesses, our dangerous "tepid" walk, lets us know we will lose the battle if we don't "beat the pirate within us." His basic call for the training of radical Christian leaders today, based on Paul's ageless counsel to his leader-disciple, moves me to my knees again and to that very action he proposes we need to take.

Alf Cooper
Archdeacon
Iglesia Anglicana de Chile+

Reading Ed Hird is an investment in a sharper mind and a closer walk with God. His inspiring stories and commentary are instructive, entertaining, and so welcome. I'm not sure the Church needs anything more badly than healthy leaders who love and follow Jesus. So don't buy a copy of this book. Buy six copies and give them to friends, relatives and complete strangers.

Phil Callaway
author and host of Laugh Again radio

Restoring Health: Body, Mind and Spirit by Ed Hird is a one-of-a-kind. It weaves ex-pert theological commentary on the book of Titus; comprehensive insights regard-ing our triune nature as humans; as well as firsthand observations of the Island of Crete where Titus was based—and did I mention pirates??? This is not your typical commentary—this is one you'll WANT to read.

Tor Constantino
MBA, former journalist
and bestselling author

As a former personal trainer and health enthusiast I believe that prayer and Bible study are to the spirit what exercise and healthy eating are to the body. Rev. Ed Hird shows how we can embrace this holistically healthy life through the verse-by-verse commentary of the book of Titus. He opens up Paul's letter and takes us on an interesting journey of discovery combined with history lessons. I recommend this book as an instruction manual for the next generation of healthy leaders.

Kimberley Payne
Author of *Women of Strength* and *Fit for Faith – 7 weeks to improved spiritual and physical health*
www.kimberleypayne.com

In reading Ed's latest book, *Restoring Health: Body, Mind and Spirit*, I found that I didn't want to put it down. In his winsome manner, Ed confronts the lure of pirate booty, treasures of the wide road that beckons to unsuspecting travelers. In mining the depths of Titus with rich insight, Ed presents to us "modern-day-pirates," a challenge for developing Godly character and leadership, for becoming whole in body, mind and spirit; for becoming holy unto the Lord. Thank you, Ed, for lighting a brilliant beacon for our journey.

Keith Bird
editor and webmaster for Order of St Luke
Communications in Canada.

Restoring Health: Body, Mind and Spirit
Published by His Publishing Group

Library of Congress Control Number: 2014948944

ISBN 978-0-9782022-1-7

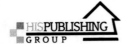

HIS Publishing Group
1402 Corinth St., Suite 131
Dallas, TX 75225

HIS Publishing Group is a division of Human Improvement Specialists, llc.
For information visit www.hispubg.com or contact publisher at info@hispubg.com

Book design by Wm. Glasgow Design, Abbotsford, BC.
Front cover photograph is courtesy Bob Grahame
Printed in the United States of America

Contents

1: Strengthening Healthy Leaders (Titus Chapter 1) 19

2: Strengthening the Generations (Titus Chapter 2) 57

3: Strengthening Other's Health (Titus Chapter 3) 71

Dedication

This book is dedicated to my favorite person Janice who has been my beloved wife for thirty-seven years so far. She is such an inspiration to me in my writing and ministry.

I would also like to thank Bill Glasgow and Larry Lube for their key roles in design and publishing services of this book.

Special thanks are due to Ginny Jaques and many others who helped me in the lengthy editing and revising process.

In Christ,
Ed Hird+

Foreword

by The Rev. Dr. J.I. Packer

Think of Shakespeare. Each of his plays is distinctive, having its own character and plot. Some of them are grander than others. But they all have the tang, so to speak, of Shakespeare, and it is hard to imagine any of them being written by anyone else.

So with Paul's letters. Each is different, and they are not all equally weighty. But in each, we meet the same person: the apostle who lives under the authority of his risen Lord and Saviour, and of the divine message of which he has been made trustee; the teacher who calls constantly for faith in the truth of that message and in its Christ, God-man, sin-bearer, conqueror of death, discipler and coming judge; the pastor who insists that faith must show itself and unshakeable hope and conscientious, law-keeping love. In all Paul's letters, the flavour of his gospel is steady, sweet and strong, and that is as true of Titus as it is of any.

Titus is sometimes dismissed as a dull, possibly non-Pauline rehash of things that Paul says more vividly elsewhere, notably in his letters to his prize protégé Timothy. But such a verdict is unperceptive, not to say perverse. Titus was Paul's second deputy after Timothy, and Paul had left him on the island of Crete to finish setting in order the congregations of first-generation converts there. Was this a tough task? Yes. Cretan culture, so it appears, was casual, morally sloppy, undisciplined, self-indulgent, and self-absorbed. It is true that in his letter to Titus, Paul spells out Christian essentials in a somewhat laborious way, but this does not mean that he doubts the adequacy of Titus' grasp of the Christian basics; what it shows, rather, is that he is going over in his own mind the full and forthright terms in which the fundamentals needed to be impressed on the Christian believers. Equally forthright statements, be it said, to young churches and church plants are sometimes needed today.

Ed Hird is a working pastor, a gospel veteran whose bailiwick for many years has arguably had something of Crete in it. He recognizes the realism of this letter, and his exposition brings it out. I heartily commend what he has written.

Dr. J.I. Packer,
Board of Governors' Professor of Theology at Regent College;
Prolific author, including *Knowing God*,
Recently named by *Time* magazine as among
the 25 most influential evangelicals in America

Preface

We have all been painfully stuck. Being at a key transition-point in our lives, we do not know how to move forward, finding ourselves immobilized.[2] I have been there many times. My perfectionism makes it worse. A key turning point for me was when as I attended a Leadership Conference at the University of Kent in England.[3] Walking into a seminar, God 'whispered' to me that I would be receiving a message. The Rev Freda Meadows suddenly called me out of the crowd and gave me a specific prophetic message, saying:

> You don't need to run in keeping up with others. Enter into God's rest. Keep your eye on the finishing line which is Him. You will be moving into new things, having words of knowledge. You will be gifted in this area. You are in an apprenticeship time at present. You will disciple others. You are a man of God's Word, things of the Kingdom. You are a person of vision, a long-range visionary. God is going to put you in a key place and you will find yourself training and discipling others.[4]

I had no idea how powerfully God was going to use the 1998 Pre-Lambeth Leadership Conference. Most of us as North American Anglicans were still stuck in the 'inside strategy' mindset. Being conflict-avoiders, we were going to 'fix' the North American Anglican churches while still inside the old institution. This virus of institutionalism can slip inside the mind of even the most sincere believer, turning us toxic. It is so easy to become the hollow, stuffed men of TS Eliot's poem: "We are the hollow men. We are the stuffed men Leaning together..."[5] We Canadians were still quite 'gung-ho' at the Canterbury Leadership Conference, but the Americans were unusually quiet. They lacked their usual American 'get-up-and-go' attitude. When Americans go quiet, you can tell that something is up.

At the official Canadian night, Bishop Eddie Marsh of Central Newfoundland invited the Americans to come up and share. I will never forget how our American colleagues Bishop Alex Dickson and Dr. (now Bishop) John Rodgers stood up and repented to our African colleagues for the shame that the USA had brought on the Anglican Church, and for Bishop John Spong's castigating African Anglicans as just one step out of animism and witchcraft.[6]

> "(Bishop Spong) has insulted you. We are ashamed for him; we are ashamed for ourselves. We ask your forgiveness and we assure you that he does not speak for us."[7]

Hundreds of African bishops and clergy spontaneously flocked forward and hugged the Americans, weeping and declaring God's forgiveness. Todd Wetzel of *Anglicans United* said that 'this was one of the American Church's finest moments in decades.' This prophetic action of repentance and forgiveness was a new beginning for Anglican Christians around the world.

I am convinced that we are not to despise prophecy, and that the prophetic gift is still in operation today. Prophecy does not just address the global picture. It can also address our personal situations, even regarding writing a book. Through prayer, I have received very clear direction about the topic of this current book.[8] Pushing through our toxic stuckness is key to restoring health, and key to strengthening a new generation of healthy leaders.

The purpose of prophecy is to encourage, build, and strengthen.[9] Yes, all prophecies have to be tested. As children of the New Covenant, we only prophesy in part.[10] Prophecies help me push through my 'what ifs' and 'if onlys'. In the 21st century, a sensitive use of the gifts of prophecy and exhortation will be essential to getting unstuck, to becoming a healthier and more Christlike leader. As Paul said to Timothy, by following prophecies made about us, we leaders more effectively 'fight the good fight' and live out our daily lives.[11] Out of these prophetic encounters, I have become convinced that North America desperately needs to recover from its toxicity, and that the key to restoring its health is found in strengthening a new generation of holistically healthy leaders, as illustrated in the person of Titus.

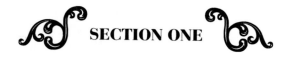

SECTION ONE

Strengthening Healthy Leaders

(Titus Chapter 1)

Who was Titus? What do we know about him? Why does he matter so much? Titus is referred to twelve times by name in the New Testament, first appearing in Jerusalem with Paul and Barnabas.[12] Unlike Timothy, Titus as a Greek was left uncircumcised by Paul in order to demonstrate freedom in Christ for the Gentiles.[13] Titus was the quintessential healthy leader. Only healthy leaders reproduce healthy leaders.

That is why Titus was sent by Paul to the island of Crete which had been swarming with pirates for the previous 800 years.[14] Even Homer's Odyssey talks about Cretan pirates. The book of Titus makes no overall sense when piracy is ignored. Pirates are the quintessential unhealthy leaders. Titus produced healthy leaders from unhealthy pirates. There are remarkable parallels between Paul's letters to Timothy and Titus.[15] They both contain unique words not found in Paul's other letters, like godliness (eusebia), soundness/health (hygenia), and self-control/sober (sophronein). Some commentators like Friedrich Schleiermacher dismissed these unique words as inauthentic, bourgeois and second-century.[16] Paul's words however make total sense when seen in light of the distinctive challenges of a toxic pirate island becoming godly, healthy and sober minded. The book of Titus is Paul's health instruction manual to unhealthy pirates. The historian Eusebius described the Pastoral Epistles as 'well known and undisputed'. No one in early church history ever doubted that Paul was the author.[17] These Pastoral Epistles are priceless treasures; they express Paul's final message of hard-won wisdom learned over many years of leadership.[18] That is why they were described as excellent and profitable for everyone.[19] There is no better health advice out there. Paul shows laser-focus in Titus and Timothy on the marks of comprehensively healthy leadership. The letter to Titus however is much shorter with only three chapters and 46 verses; In contrast the letters to Timothy involve ten chapters and 196 verses.

Paul chose Titus who had a very different personality, a different 'DNA' than Timothy. While Timothy needed a lot of cheerleading to stay motivated, Titus was self-motivated and fearless. He was the perfect mentor for unhealthy ex-pirates, as you could not intimidate or manipulate him. Titus never needed the welcome given to shy Timothy when Paul went out of his way to make sure that the Corinthians did not reject him.[20] Like a spiritual paratrooper, Titus was dropped in the middle of some of the most difficult assignments that you could imagine: to the Corinthians, the Cretans and the Dalmatians. You could describe Titus as Paul's trouble-shooter. As a 'Star-Trekker' of the first degree, Titus boldly went where others feared to tread, where others had never been before.

Who in their right mind would want to be sent to a toxic island where everyone was a pirate, including the grandmothers, grandsons, and everyone in between? Who would want to be sent to an island where all islanders were liars, evil brutes and lazy gluttons? Titus was just the man for the job. He did not flinch. He did not moan or complain. When Paul said 'jump,' Titus never questioned. He just said 'how high?'" He was a true pioneer leader who has inspired tens of thousands of pioneering leaders for the last two thousand years. Titus taught toxic Cretan pirates how to become radically healthy: how to love, how to lay down their lives for another, how to be the faithful husband of but one wife, how to be gentle and patient. He taught the female pirates how to be best friends with their husbands and their children. This is true health. If the wisdom in the 45-sentence book of Titus can revolutionize a pirate island, it can even transform a pirate continent like North America. Signs of our North American toxicity include gun violence and the insanity of the shooters, obesity when there is no shortage of food, and a wealth of communication tools while many are no longer talking any more.

Is it a mere coincidence that the late Steve Jobs defined Apple employees as pirates, even raising a pirate flag with the Apple logo as the pirate eye-patch? It is better, said Jobs, to be a pirate than join the navy.[21] In the 1999 movie *Pirates of Silicon Valley,* Jobs accused Bill Gates of ripping him off by producing the *Microsoft Windows* mouse-based graphical user interface. Gates, the wealthiest person on earth, memorably said to his outraged fellow pirate Steve Jobs: "we both had this rich neighbor named Xerox and I broke into his house to steal the TV set and found out that you had already stolen it."[22] Ironically Jobs loved to quote Picasso's comment: "Good artists copy. Great artists steal." So do great pirates.

Besides Crete, Titus was also sent to the wild Corinthian Christians who were extreme in terms of hyper-spirituality and sexual confusion. They too were a pirate church, much like our North American Church culture. In 2 Corinthians 7:6, Paul comments that "God, who comforts the downcast, comforted us by the coming of Titus…" Paul wrote two of his most challenging letters to the out-of-control Corinthians. William Barclay, referring to Titus in Corinth, said that:

> There are two kinds of people. There are the people who can make a bad situation worse, and there are the people who can bring order out of chaos and peace out of strife.[23]

This orderly, peaceful Titus was a man of challenge and a man of comfort. He was one of those unique leaders who had the grace to be both strong and gentle, compassionate and discerning.[24] Titus had unusual tact, possessing great leadership gifts.[25] Paul knew that Titus, as a man of financial integrity, wouldn't run off with the checkbook. Because of Titus' radical honesty,

Paul could assign him to sort out the Corinthians financially and also safely bring the generous gift to the hurting Jerusalem believers.

Titus was a first-century go-getter. He reminds me of my father, Ted Hird, who always gets the job done. At one of my father's retirements, his company, *Microtel*, gave him a statue of a horse in memory of my father's billing the company for a dead horse. Working in Newfoundland for three months with the snowy roads sometimes impassable, my father hired a farmer's horse to drag the telecommunications equipment up the hill. The microwave tower was finally finished, but the horse died. Titus-like leaders make things happen against impossible odds.

In the twelve-step movement, we are told that anyone can become healthy if they are willing to become rigorously honest.[26] Titus was a person of deep convictions. He stood for the truth, even when it cost him deeply. Titus was loyal to Paul and his leadership team in a way that we seldom see in our individualistic 'me-first' pirate culture.[27]

There is much distrust of leadership by twenty-first century people who have been hurt by abuses of power or by inept dithering. As a baby-boomer, I acknowledge that our generation has made many tragic mistakes. We have too often acted toxically like Cretan pirates. Titus was a healthy leader who would not exploit you and did not waste your time in bureaucratic nonsense. That is why the apostle Paul poured his life into Titus, and entrusted him with his most difficult assignments. I have sometimes regretted my voting for certain politicians or my appointing particular leaders. Paul never regretted having put his trust in Titus' leadership. In an age of many regrets, Titus is a symbol of hope for healthy leadership in the twenty-first century.

With the huge global changes happening, the need for Tituses has never been greater. A key solution to our North American toxicity is rediscovering Titus, the epitome of integrated healthy leadership. Titus was a church planter par excellence who planted significantly healthy churches by identifying and training indigenous leaders in every one of the over hundred Cretan cities.[28] The book of Titus gives you the keys to healthy churches, healthy families and healthy lives.

Titus was an enthusiastic self-starter who showed remarkable initiative, thriving in challenging settings. This is why Paul said, "Titus not only welcomed our appeal, but he is coming to you with much enthusiasm and on his own initiative"[29]. Titus was a passionately missional leader. He thought and acted like a missionary, reproducing that same missionary zeal in all of his disciples. He had an eagerness and courage that was contagious.[30] So many churches in North America are sadly self-centered. We are too often more survival-oriented than mission-focused. Imagine what would happen if every congregation had a Titus in their midst. Imagine what would happen if tens of thousands of healthy Tituses were strengthened and released throughout the pirate continent of North America and to the ends of the earth.

That is our challenge: to send forth Tituses all across North America and worldwide who can plant many comprehensively healthy churches, churches that are immunized against deception and false teaching. The future is released when we own up to our mistakes as the Church, and find a new way to move forward. It is time, as Jesus recommended, to pull the logs out of our own pirate eyes and to invest in a new generation of healthy leaders.

Because of the moral and spiritual confusion being sown in Crete by false teachers, Paul's key emphasis to Titus again and again was holistic health/soundness: healthy faith, healthy doctrine, healthy love, and healthy endurance. Health for Paul was not just physical. Paul insisted on health in every area of Titus's life as he impacted the Cretans. The very Greek word for both health and soundness is 'hygiaino' ὑγιαίνω from which we get the modern term 'hygiene'. Many people do not realize that soundness and health are the same biblical concept. When a heart is healthy, the doctor says that it is sound. The book of Titus was not merely about healthy/sound doctrine. Health for Paul was holistic, embracing our whole life in body, mind and spirit. That is why Paul prayed in 1 Thessalonians 5:23: "May your whole spirit, soul/psyche and body be kept blameless at the coming of our Lord Jesus Christ."[31]

Both terms 'health' and 'heal' comes from the West Germanic word 'hailaz' for wholeness. The Concise Oxford Dictionary defines 'heal' as 'restore to health, become sound or whole'. The book of Titus calls us to become whole people – in mind, body, and spirit – who embody the whole gospel. So often we North American pirates are toxically fragmented in areas of our lives. We need the Great Physician to give us a full check-up to determine whether our lives, our marriages and families, our churches and communities are sound and healthy. Many of us are out of balance in our health emphasis, neglecting either the body, the mind or the spirit. The ancient gnostic heresy caused people to reject the physical world in favour of abstract spirituality. I have seen far too many good church people gnostically neglecting their bodies and minds. Too many good people have bought the lie that they can eat anything they want and not bother to exercise. The Bible says that our health choices have consequences. We reap as we sow. People who neglect their bodies lose the ability to travel cross-culturally as they get older. People who neglect their minds go stale and have nothing worth saying. People who neglect their spirits go shallow and self-absorbed. Healthy leaders embrace their bodies, minds and spirits for Christ's sake.

TITUS 1:1 *"Paul, a servant of God and an apostle of Jesus Christ for the faith of God's elect and the knowledge of the truth that leads to godliness."*

Healthy leadership leads to holistic godliness in body, mind and spirit. Godliness was never supposed to be merely spiritual. It is practical and life-changing. Paul begins this 46-verse letter with a rather dense introduction, emphasizing both who he is as a leader and what he aims to accomplish.[32] Paul has an amazing way of holding apparent paradoxes in dynamic tension. He is both a servant and an apostle. Apostolic leadership is about being healthy shepherds who can both defend sheep from wolves and bind up the wounded sheep. For Paul, both the faith of God's elect and the knowledge of the truth are bottom line issues. Many North Americans split faith from knowledge, often seeing faith as superstitious and irrelevant to health. Knowledge of the truth needs to be understood holistically, as involving the whole person in their body, mind and spirit. Pirate cultures and pirate churches suppress truth and minimize its importance. Yet truth matters and potentially changes everything. It is not merely abstract and theoretical. Truth is both conceptual and experiential. This truth is meant to be known both objectively and subjectively.

Why does faith need to go hand-in-hand with knowledge? Without faith and knowledge, there is no godliness, no holiness, and no health. Faith and knowledge are Siamese twins. Nothing is true, nothing is faithful, if it does not lead to healthy godliness, to Christ-likeness. Truth is a person. Jesus is the embodiment of all truth, all godliness, and all health. In the book of Titus, godliness and healthiness are interchangeable concepts. Many North Americans tend to artificially split godliness from health. Godliness belongs in a sanctuary, while health is found at the gym. The book of Titus holds them together in dynamic tension. Godliness is biblical healthiness. Godliness is meant to make you more, not less human. That is why Titus was instructed to ground the ex-pirate Cretans in both healthy doctrine and godly living.

The late Dr John Stott said that the most important thing in life is Christ-likeness.[33] To be biblically healthy or sound is to be Christlike. Because Jesus Christ was the most human, he was also the most holistically healthy. Jesus would have been very physically fit, hiking everywhere he went. One of his favorite places to pray was on mountain tops. Twice Jesus physically overturned money changers' tables, casting them out of the temple. He certainly was mentally and spiritually fit, able to engage creatively with some of the greatest intellectuals and spiritual leaders in the Middle East.

Integrated health and godliness are apostolic priorities. The book of Titus gives us a first-hand understanding of what it means to be one holy, catholic and apostolic church. Our apostolic heritage of healthy Christ-likeness trumps our toxic pirate heritage. Where you are heading apostolically is more important than where you came from.

TITUS 1:2 *"a faith and knowledge resting on the hope of eternal life, which God, who does not lie, promised before the beginning of time…"*

When I lose hope as a leader, I lose energy. Faith and knowledge rest upon and depend upon hope. Restoring health is rooted in everlasting and unshakable hope. Biblical hope is all about choosing life and health in the midst of death. Hope is grounded in God's covenant promises. Why trust God? Because God, unlike the rest of us, cannot lie when he makes a promise. Our Father is utterly trustworthy. If God were a liar, we would be in serious trouble. There would be nothing that we can trust. The God in whom we believe shapes who we become as holistically healthy leaders. If our God is truthful, we become more truthful. If our God is a liar, we become liars. Our view of God is the truest thing about us as leaders. As Bishop NT Wright put it, the (Greek) gods were unpredictable, potentially dangerous, and even malevolent.[34] Malevolent gods make malevolent leaders. A godly, healthy God makes godly, healthy leaders. The God who cannot lie produced ex-pirates in Crete who could no longer lie. This change would have been shocking and revolutionary. Their newfound honesty changed everything. Have you ever felt betrayed by people that you have voted for? Imagine what a newfound honesty could do in restoring godliness and health to our North American businesses and governments.

Thank God for wives that are holistically health-conscious. They help us recover from our unhealthy pirate tendencies. My wife Janice cares for me enough to honestly tell me when I am being unhealthy. She shows her love by encouraging me to go to the gym, eat healthy food, take vitamins, and have a daily quiet time. Restoring holistic health requires that I practice what I preach. It is not enough for me to gnostically focus on the spiritual and neglect my body, God's very own temple. It is too easy for me to be a health-conscious hypocrite. Most North Americans already conceptually know how to become more healthy. We genuinely want to and intend to be more healthy. The road to destruction is too often paved with good intentions. Owning a gym pass doesn't guarantee that I actually go to the gym. Sometimes I have been tempted to not regularly get to the gym so that I have more time to write about regularly going to the gym. Satan's plausible lie is that I do not have time to be holistically healthy. The North Shore, where I live and work, is obsessed with busyness. Busyness is often the mortal enemy of being comprehensively healthy. As a Spanish proverb puts it, a man too busy to take care of his health is like a mechanic too busy to take care of his tools.

Going to the gym two to three times a week for the past fourteen years is part of my 'walking the walk' of holistic health. I feel healthier and younger now than a decade ago, having lost twenty-five pounds in the process, going from 180 to 155 pounds. Rather than potentially needing to take medication, my cholesterol and blood pressure are now healthy. The Good Book tells us that even the youth grow weary, but they that wait on the Lord shall renew and restore their strength, rising up with wings like eagles, running and not being weary, walking and not fainting.[35]

Part of what drove me to the gym was being rear-ended by a taxi. I started going for various treatments to loosen up my neck and shoulders, but nothing seemed to really last. The neck spasms and headaches had a nasty habit of sapping a lot of my energy needed for work and family. Finally my chiropractor Dr. Paul Wiggins, while adjusting my aching back, said to me: "You need a personal trainer". My immediate reaction was to try to graciously change the subject. Paul was very persistent in a kindly way, and the next thing I knew, I was meeting with a personal trainer for six sessions, paid for by our auto insurance company.

I have been involved in many sports and exercise programs over the years. Sooner or later I usually would push it too far and too fast, and injure myself. So many boomers are injuring themselves through overdoing exercise that this condition is being called 'boomeritis.'[36] Once injured and 'humbled', I often thought twice before 'getting back in the ring'. I was once very close to having neck surgery after a pinched nerve sent burning pains down my left arm, continually waking me up in the middle of the night. I couldn't type or play guitar with my left hand. The neck surgeon, whom I met with, gave me the worst case scenario. It was very scary. Thanks to those sessions with my personal trainer and my physiotherapist, I am once again typing, playing guitar, and working out at the gym. Having finally learned how to pace myself, I rarely injure myself now. I have learnt that the secret to virtually all the gym equipment is going 'one step at a time'. Patience, while not my strongest characteristic, is definitely a virtue in the weight room!

Benjamin Franklin once said: "Health is man's best wealth."[37] People often spend their health to obtain wealth, only to spend their wealth to obtain health. As Boomers are aging, we are sometimes understandably concerned that we may be going backwards in health rather than moving forward. Many seem to have fatalistically lost hope. But must aging always be a downward spiral? The God, who cannot lie, promises to renew our youth like an eagle.[38] What I am hearing from the Lord is "Do not give up on yourself. Do not give up on your dreams of finishing well. Why not choose to be fit? Why not choose to be healthier?"

Physical fitness is good, but by itself only goes so far. The well-known Washington DC author Mark Batterson twittered: "In my experience, physical disciplines like exercise and spiritual disciplines like prayer feed off each other."[39] Health is elusive. We are our own worst enemies. We want to be holistically healthy. Yet we make choices such as too much food, too little exercise, and self-medication that cripple us and send us in the wrong direction. As a local Recreation Centre poster put it, "The hardest thing about exercise is to start doing it." Edward Stanley said it well: "Those who think they will not have time for bodily exercise will sooner or later have to find time for illness."[40] That is why Jesus asked: "Do you want to be well?" Why do we resist getting well? Why do we talk the health talk and not walk the health walk? Why are we so often reluctant to give up excess sugar and salt? Why are we so often tempted to just let nature take its course? So many people die before their time. As Mark Twain put it, most men die at age 27. We just bury them at 72.[41] Pirates were notorious for being unhealthy and dying young. My passion is to help a new generation of comprehensively healthy leaders discover and rediscover Jesus as the Great Physician who renews our youth like an eagle.

Healthy hearts and healthy minds lead to healthy lives, healthy choices and healthy families. John said, "Dear friend, I pray that you may enjoy good health and that all things may go well with you, even as your soul is getting along well." (3 John 2) Integral health comes through the power of the Holy Spirit. As Dr. E. Stanley Jones put it:

> The Spirit of God is health… A health tendency takes possession of us. We think health. We breathe health; we are health & we give health.[42]

If the toxic Cretan pirates can become healthy, anyone can become healthy, even North Americans. Dr. Brene Brown, whose TED talk has been seen by over sixteen million people, said that we in North America "are the most in-debt, obese, addicted and medicated adult cohort in (our) history."[43] The book of Titus sets the tone for the early Christians to be passionate about being holistically healthy. It was standard practice to pray for the sick in the power of the Holy Spirit. Colin Cross comments that the early Church:

> ...saw the Christ as a physician, the Church as a hospital, the sacraments as medication and orthodoxy as 'a medicine chest against heresy'.[44]

I will never forget the night that Lee Grady, former Editor of Charisma Magazine, prophesied about St. Simon's NV being a well-spring of healing with healing teams being raised up for body, soul and spirit restoration. Every worship service at St. Simon's NV, whether traditional or contemporary, has a team ready to pray for healing. I believe that this book is part of the fulfillment of Lee Grady's prophecy.[45] Imagine how wellsprings of healing, Titus communities, might revolutionize our toxic North American pirate culture.

Searching for health in a Mediterranean paradise

So how does a new generation of North American leaders become more holistically healthy? What does this look like? As part of writing this book, my wife and I flew to Crete where we found out that countless Cretans have been radically transformed by Titus' whole gospel of Life over death. Cretans today remember him as 'Bishop Titus' or 'St. Titus/ Hagio Tito', even crediting him with the absence of venomous snakes on the island! We took time to view Titus' head at Hagio Tito Church which was returned by the Venetians to Crete in 1966. The historian Eusebius tells us that Titus returned to Crete and served as a bishop there until his old age.[46] In the fourteenth-century "Revolt of St Titus" against the Venetians, Crete even became known as the Republic of St Titus.[47] We found the Cretan people very hospitable, especially Fr. Makarios Grinezakis, the official preacher for the Orthodox Church of Crete. Fr. Makarios was a priest, medical doctor, monk, radio station director, and principal of their Cretan Seminary.[48]

You will remember how Paul in Titus 1:12 quoted the sixth century B.C. Cretan prophet, Epimenides: "All Cretans are liars, evil brutes, lazy gluttons". And to make matters worse, Paul added: 'this testimony is true!' Imagine if Paul had said that all Canadians or all Americans are liars, evil brutes, and lazy gluttons. Canadians most likely would be deeply offended and hurt. But not first Century Cretans. Piracy was how they and their ancestors had made an 'honorable' living for as long as they could remember. It was who they were, the very core of their identity and self-image. They had been pirates for over 800 years and were proud of their gifts for lying, violence and gluttony. Even the youngest child, going on Disney-land's Pirates of the Caribbean ride, knows that lying, violence and gluttony is what pirates do best. Errol Flynn, or Johnny Depp who played the charmingly deceptive Captain Jack Sparrow of the movie series *Pirates of the Caribbean,* would have been right at home in first-century Crete. Putting Hollywood fantasy aside, "a pirate's life was invariably nasty, brutish and short."[49] The miracle is that through the 'renewing of the Holy Spirit' (Titus 3:5), deceitful, violent, addicted buccaneers became trustworthy, peaceful, and sober. The Cretan miracle of healthy godliness can become the North American miracle.

Pirates are waiting for us around every North American corner. The Concise Oxford Dictionary defines pirates as marauders. The root Greek term for pirates (*peirao*) means assault.[50] After dropping my wife at work, I walked by *Martin Marine Boat Hardware Store* on the way to working out at the local gym. In the hardware window, I saw pirate paraphernalia galore: pirate clocks, pirate flags, pirate cups, pirate chests, pirate washcloths, pirate scarf's, pirate pencils, pirate wallets, pirate baseball caps, and even pirate hats. Pirate paraphernalia is big business! Atlanta Georgia is reportedly cashing in on this new fad with a proposed Pirate Museum.[51] There are already Pirate Museums in Massachusetts, North Carolina and Florida, including two in Key West. Some claim that piracy is humanity's third oldest profession, after prostitution and medicine.[52] Mark Twain playfully wrote: "Now and then we had a hope that if we lived and were good, God would permit us to be pirates."[53] It was a family tradition, said Twain, that his ancestors were Elizabethan pirates, back when it was a respectable trade.[54] Many of us fondly remember how Twain had Tom Sawyer and Huckleberry Finn run away in an attempt to become pirates on the Mississippi. Perhaps we North Americans are more like pirates at heart than we might want to admit.

While some are tempted to think of pirates as relics of a colonial past, news about a $35 million dollar ransom demanded by Somalian pirates reminds us that piracy is alive and well in many parts of the world.[55] Rather than just using a cutlass, they employ automatic weapons, rocket-propelled grenades, and shoulder-launched ground-to-air missiles. It is estimated that Somalian pirates bring in an annual booty of over fifty million dollars. Every year over 16,000 ships pass by the Somalian coast, one of the world's busiest shipping areas linking Asia to Europe. You may remember how the Somalian pirates were brash enough to take over a Saudi supertanker carrying over 100 million dollars of crude oil. Imagine if Paul, instead of sending Titus to Crete, had sent him to Somalia and told him to plant over one hundred indigenous churches among the Somalian coastal pirates.

TITUS 1:3 *"...and at his appointed season he brought his word to light through the preaching entrusted to me by the command of God our Savior..."*

Does the cross have anything to do with becoming a healthy leader? Titus in Crete was preaching about the cross to self-declared practicing pirates, people who easily could have been indifferent or hostile. Yet these pirates eagerly embraced it. To many people in North America, God is a nuisance, an interference in our busy lives. "Do not tell me what to do with my life", they may say. Many others have decided that the Christian faith is unimportant and not worth paying attention. Dr. E. Stanley Jones commented that "it is easier to meet opposition than it is to meet indifference."[56] Indifference is a worse sin than atheism, because it is so unresponsive. It treats Jesus like he does not matter. Paul talks about the foolishness of preaching, the scandal of the good news. This radical message of Jesus Christ hanging on a tree is the wisdom and power of God.[57] Only the cross can transform hardened Cretan and North American pirates into holistically healthy leaders. Only God's Word can bring light into our pirate hearts.

TITUS 1:4 *"To Titus, my true son in our common faith: Grace and peace from God the Father and Christ Jesus our Savior."*

Healthy leadership is about strengthening our spiritual sons and daughters in our common faith. Our faith is either 'common' or it is not real. Although Titus was not Jewish, Paul identified him in the same way he addressed Timothy as his true son. Perhaps Paul had led both to Christ. One of the reasons I love the Anglican Book of Common Prayer is that it is common, shared, and not merely individualistic. Privatism is a toxic disease that is at war with our common faith. There is no such thing as a genuine Christian faith that we make up on our own. Far too often, the gods of our own private understanding are really the idols of our hearts. Paul prayerfully extended grace and peace to Titus, which Douglas Milnes calls "the beginning and end of Christian life."[58] At the very heart of being healthy, of being sound is the gift of grace and peace. These two qualities are essential to surviving and thriving as ex-pirates. Do any of us need less grace and less peace in our busy lives?

Like Israel, Crete gets into your soul. You do not forget it. Crete was full of grace and peace. Being in Crete was like being in one huge Greek restaurant. My wife Janice and I loved the food. The tone, culture, and music are very soothing and captivating, reflecting the beauty of Crete and the unbreakable spirit of its people.[59] Dr. Philip Towner commented that Crete's "history is that of an island located well for sea trade, a home for piracy, the famous hundred cities, and much inter-city fighting." [60] Crete is a 152-mile long island, the fifth largest island in the Mediterranean, ranging from 7 to 32 miles in width. As the largest of the Greek Islands (3,219 square miles[61]), it has mountains up to 8,000 feet, composed mostly of bare limestone, honeycombed with caves and liable to earthquake.[62] These caves "formed the first shrines and cult centers, provided refuge from pirates, hideouts for bandits and revolutionaries in the uprisings of the eighteenth and nineteenth centuries, and for partisans during the Second World War"[63]

Most of Crete's 500,000+ people live in the north part of Crete. The fictional 'Zorba the Greek', from the Cretan writer Nikos Kazantzakis, turned out to be 'born' in Crete. While many Greeks look to Crete as the most authentic of the Greek Islands, Cretans rarely refer to themselves as Greeks.[64]

It was fascinating to visit the Cretan Palace of Knossos, where the Bronze Age Minoan culture emerged from 2600 BC to 1400 BC. Because Greek, and indeed European, civilization can be traced back to Crete, there are reportedly over 2,000 scholars and archeologists on Crete.[65] Even the name Europe comes from Princess Europa who was the wife of the Cretan King Asterios. Cretans believed that Crete, rather than Olympus, was the true birthplace of Greek religion and culture. They even taught that Zeus himself, the 'man become god', was buried in Crete.[66]

I had no idea before I began this Cretan pilgrimage that the Cretans are the direct ancestors of the biblical Philistines. Michael Griffiths comments that from Knossos:

> "the 'Sea Peoples' (including the Philistines) migrated to the Eastern end of the Mediterranean. After being repulsed by Egypt, they built five city states (Gath, Ashkelon, Ashdod, Ekron, and Gaza) on the coastal plain...."[67]

In Amos 9:7, the Lord says 'Did I not bring Israel up from Egypt, the Philistines from Caphtor and the Arameans from Kir?" Caphtor is the Hebrew name for the island of Crete.[68] The Kerethites of King David's bodyguard (2 Samuel 15:18) were native-born Cretan mercenaries[69]

Crete has a long history of being conquered by many other nations, including the Romans, Turks, Egyptians, Arabs, and most recently the Nazis.[70] The Venetians were in charge from 1204 to 1669 when the Turks took over after the siege of Candia (1648–1669). The Cretans remember this as the longest recorded siege in modern history. The loss of Candia was devastating to Europe because they lost access to Candia's candy and honey.[71] Crete has a particularly favorable climate for bee-keeping. Losing Candia meant that Europe's sweet tooth had to be satisfied by Cuban cane sugar and India's delicacies. The term 'candy' comes from the Cretian town Candia (modern-day Heraklion) where the sweets were produced. Some of the most well-preserved archeological findings at the Palace of Knossos are the beautiful honey pots. You may remember how Edmund in the Narnia Chronicles was seduced by the white witch through his love of Turkish Delight, which was just a post-1669 name for Cretan honey, mixed with meringue, almonds and nuts.[72]

Plato tells us that such candied fruits were popular sacrificial gifts to the Greek gods.[73] Cretan honey was also needed for embalming and used in many temples and sanctuaries dedicated to the rites for the Dead.[74] When Alexander the Great died in Babylon in 323 BC, he was preserved in honey.[75]

Right near our Hotel Castello in the capital City of Heraklion, we saw the statue of Captain Michael Korakis, the 1821 liberator of Crete from Turkish rule. Several bishops were martyred during this uprising, and twenty percent of the Cretan population perished. Britain decided that Crete was not allowed to join Greece, fearing that Crete would either once again become a center of piracy or a Russian naval base. So Crete was reconquered by Egypt, a vassal of Turkey.[76]

TITUS 1:5 *"The reason I left you in Crete was that you might put in order what was left unfinished and appoint elders in every town, as I directed you."*

Healthy leadership is about finishing well. Many baby boomers are realizing that there is much unfinished in their lives, much that still needs to be set in order. You will notice that Paul got right to the point with Titus: "the reason I left you in Crete". When Paul sent Titus to Crete, he was not 'starting from scratch'. We know from the book of Acts that some Cretans were present and filled with the Holy Spirit on the Day of Pentecost.[77] That is why Paul was not speaking to Titus about starting from nothing but rather "straightening out what is left unfinished".[78] Rome was not built in a day. Neither was the healthy new Cretan Church. There is no lasting quick fix when transforming toxic pirates into healthy leaders. Strengthening a new generation of Tituses takes time. Yet this is the key to finishing well. As John Calvin put it,

> Building a church is no easy task and cannot be completed in a moment... (Paul) was naturally exceptionally talented, he never grew tired in all his work, and yet he confesses that he left the work half done....it takes more than just a year or two to restore a fallen church.[79]

Crete was a port of call on any eastbound voyage from Italy. We know that Paul as a prisoner on his way to Rome landed at Fair Havens on the south coast of Crete.[80] So there was a significant Cretan connection to Paul that the Cretans remember even two thousand years later.

From the ranks of ex-pirates, Titus was commissioned by Paul to recruit and strengthen healthy indigenous leaders. This is our North American challenge in the twenty-first century. There is much to be straightened out, much left unfinished. Many of us, particularly those who are faithful Anglican Christians, are starting again from scratch. Many of us have counted all loss for the sake of following Christ (Philippians 3:8).

Without knowing where we have come from, we do not know where we are going. We must face our painful North American pirate heritage if we are to give truly healthy leadership. In CS Lewis' *Prince Caspian* story, Aslan tells us where the Telmarines, including Prince Caspian, came from:

> Many years ago in that world (the world of Adam's sons), in a deep sea of that world which is called the South Sea, a shipload of pirates were driven by storm on an island. And there they did as pirates would: killed the natives and took the native women for wives, and made palm wine, and drank and were drunk, and lay in the shade of the palm trees, and woke up and quarreled, and sometimes killed one another.[81]

Prince Caspian was embarrassed by his pirate heritage saying: "I was wishing that I was from a more noble lineage." "You come of the Lord Adam and the Lady Eve," said Aslan. "And that is both honour enough to erect the head of the poorest beggar, and shame enough to bow the shoulders of the greatest emperor on earth. Be content."[82] The embarrassing truth about each of us is that we are all Telmarines, we are all pirates, yet we are all sons and daughters of Lord Adam and Lady Eve. We are all made in God's image, and we are all sinners worthy of death, for whom Christ died. The Cretans are not the only ex-pirates out there.

TITUS 1:6 *"the husband of but one wife"*

One of the greatest challenges for the Cretan ex-pirates was how to develop healthy marriages, built on harmony and tenderness. It would be a foreign concept to them: "husband of but one wife??" The famous Pirate Captain Blackbeard was a firm believer in marriage. Some say that he had fourteen wives in different ports. Monogamy in our fragmented North American culture is often dismissed as impractical and too controlling. Yet God used biblical marriage to transform the relational chaos of the pirate island of Crete. Healthy leaders need healthy marriages. A healthy marriage between one man and one woman is God's better idea. Biblical marriage is worth sacrificing for. That is why I recently completed a Doctorate, focusing on strengthening marriages.[83] God is passionate about transforming toxic relationships.[84] Our North American relational shipwrecks can become trophies of God's mercy and restoration. What might happen if our North American society realized that God's Church has the key to marital stability and satisfaction?

TITUS 1:6 *"...a man whose children believe and are not open to the charge of being wild and disobedient."*

By the washing of new birth and renewing of the Holy Spirit, ex-pirates on Crete learned a new way of healthy parenting. As the ex-pirate parents repented of their wildness and disobedience, they modeled for their believing children a new way of living, centered in the Lordship of Jesus Christ. So often our children are the casualties of our corporate selfishness and pirate lifestyles. We need to be passionate in our post-modern culture to do everything that we can to strengthen our families. As my mentor Dr. E. Stanley Jones put it, "Be victorious in the home, and you are victorious everywhere."[85] Colossians 3:19-21 teaches that harshness to our spouse and children only serves to embitter them. God's kindness turns us from being pirates to becoming healthy family leaders. We need to pray for our pastors that their marriages and families will be a sign of hope to our very fragmented culture. As our Bishop Silas Ng has been teaching us, regular daily prayer is the key to healthy marriages, families, churches, and neighbourhoods.[86]

TITUS 1:7 *"not overbearing, not quick-tempered, not given to drunkenness."*

Pirates are famous for being overbearing and quick-tempered. Only the power of the Holy Spirit can change an overbearing pirate into a humble, Christ-like leader. It is so easy as North American pirates to be stiff-necked, stubborn, and unwilling to listen. If we think that we are always right and others are always wrong, we are in serious trouble. Our self-righteousness stinks. It is not the way of Christ. Instead of crushing the people by imposing his will, Jesus the servant-leader washes their feet with a towel and said "go and do likewise."

Thoughtless outbursts of anger are like toxic rain to marriages and family. Quick-tempered pirates are easily angered, fast to draw their sabers, quick to shoot off at the mouth. According to Benjamin Franklin, anger is never without a reason, but seldom with a good one. For Gene Getz,

> a 'quick-tempered' person easily "flies off the handle" or "loses his cool"… He often loses control and "strikes out" at others, if not physically, at least verbally.[87]

A quick-tempered Christian is 'out of control'. We all have to guard against becoming grumpy old men and women. Angry people end up being touchy and disappointed over almost everything. Unresolved anger ends in bitterness and isolation. Undealt-with anger can lead us to become "detestable, disobedient and unfit for doing anything good." (Titus 1:16) Rather than examine ourselves, anger always blames someone else: "It's not my fault. It's your fault." It is too easy to become hardened inside. During one of our worst Vancouver snowstorms, I wrote in my journal: "Remove snow while it is still soft, before it hardens. Remove offenses and unforgiveness from your heart before it hardens and gives you a heart of stone." Healthy leadership is a matter of the heart.

Self-medication through alcohol and drugs is a favorite coping technique for most pirates. Bill Wilson in the *AA Big Book* wrote:

> Resentment is the "number one" offender. It destroys more alcoholics than anything else. From it stem all form of spiritual disease, for we have been not only mentally and physically ill, we have been spiritually sick.[88]

The *Big Book* went on to say:

> If we were to live again, we had to be free of anger. The grouch and the brainstorm were not for us. They may be the dubious luxury of normal men, but for alcoholics these things are poison."[89]

I remember an AA friend telling me that becoming sober was not the hardest thing. The greatest challenge was dealing with the 'new' painful emotions that had been suppressed through all those year of over-consuming. Bill W, who had been led to Christ by the Anglican priest Dr Samuel Shoemaker, called the Holy Spirit his Higher Power. In doing this, he was drawing on Luke 24:49 where Jesus described the Holy Spirit as the "power from on high" who would clothe us as we waited on Him. Without this power from on high, this renewing of the Holy Spirit, we North American pirates are powerless to change and our lives are left unmanageable.

What is it about piracy that still captures our imagination 2,000 years later? Most of us have never met an actual pirate and yet we have a fixed idea in our mind going back to our childhood. In 1888 Robert Louis Stevenson published Treasure Island, a book that burned into our brain key ingredients of a pirate story: treasure maps and chests, wooden legs, parrots, eye patches, and 'Fifteen men on a dead man's chest.'[90] Who can forget Long John Silver and also Captain Hook of Peter Pan fame?

During Mardi Gras, pirate costumes are the most popular. Pirates symbolize the suppressed desire to rebel, to live free, to lie on a hammock in the sun, and say no to anyone's attempts to control you. It is easy to romanticize pirates, forgetting that they were ruthless men capable of savage cruelty, usually under the influence of heavy drinking. Through doing Fifth Steps with alcoholics for the past thirty-two years, I have become unshockable when people confess how they have wronged others. Why have I made the unusual step of not drinking? Because many in both sides of my family have an allergy to alcohol. At least ten percent of people should not drink, because it takes over their lives. It is not a sin to drink, but it is a sin and destructive to be drunk.[91] I have learned from over thirty-four years of ordained ministry that until someone deals with one's substance abuse issues, nothing changes. The most well-meaning new convert who refuses to deal with their alcohol and drug abuse will just go around in endless circles. That is why Alcoholics Anonymous describe alcohol as cunning, baffling and powerful.[92] Alcohol and drugs do not give control over our lives without a fight. Only the Power from on high can break this desperate cycle that is destroying so many North American families and marriages.

Perhaps one of the most famous North American ex-pirates is the *Man in Black* Johnny Cash. Alcohol and drugs ravaged his life for many years. Bono of U2 commented: "To me, Johnny Cash—with all his contradictions—was a quintessential character of the scriptures, or at least of the characters in the Bible that interested me. If God had time for these flawed characters, then God had time for me."[93] Bob Dylan said: "Listen to (Cash) and he always brings you to your senses. He rises high above all, and he'll never die

or be forgotten, even by persons not born yet—especially those persons…"
During Johnny Cash's nearly fifty years of music, he sold over ninety million albums. He learned to sing while picking cotton as an impoverished
sharecropper's son in Kingsland, Arkansas. His mother Carrie said to Johnny at age 15: "You've got a gift, JR. You're going to sing. God's got his hand
on you. You're going to carry the message of Jesus Christ."[94] Cash recorded
more than 1,500 songs including well-known hits like "A Boy named Sue",
"Folsom Prison Blues" and "Ring of Fire." Johnny Cash is the only musician
who has ever been threefold-inducted into the Songwriter's, Country Music,
and Rock and Roll Halls of Fame."[95]

More than 100 other recording artists and groups have recorded Cash's
song 'I Walk the Line." Cash commented: "I wrote 'I walk the Line' when
I was on the road in Texas in 1956, having a hard time resisting the temptation to be unfaithful to my wife back in Memphis": "I keep a close watch on
this heart of mine. I keep my eyes wide open all the time. I keep the ends
out for the tie that binds. Because you're mine, I walk the line." Cash saw 'I
walk the Line' as his first Gospel hit, because he sang it not just to his wife,
but also to God.[96]

Cash's life was often fraught with tragedy and heartbreak. "After my
brother Jack's death, said Johnny, "I felt like I'd died, too. I just didn't
feel alive. I was terribly lonely without him. I had no other friend." His
father unfairly blamed Johnny for his brother's death, saying "Too bad it
wasn't you instead of Jack."[97] Like his father before him, Johnny struggled
for many years with addiction issues. His father was never able to tell his
children that he loved them. Johnny Cash's first marriage ran aground in
the midst of workaholism and pill-popping. In Cash' autobiography, he
comments: "Touring and drugs were what I did, with the effort involved in
drugs mounting steadily as time went by." Amphetamines kept him going
without sleep, and barbiturates and alcohol knocked him out. Cash commented: "I was in and out of jails, hospitals, and car wrecks. I was a walking
vision of death, and that's exactly how I felt. I was scraping the filthy bottom of the barrel of life."[98]

He knew that he had wasted his life and drifted far from God, saying:

> I used drugs to escape and they worked pretty well when I was younger.
> But they devastated me physically and emotionally—and spiritually. That
> last one hurt so much: to put myself in such a low state that I couldn't
> communicate with God, and I wasn't even trying to call on him.[99]

In desperation, Cash decided to end his life in 1967 by crawling deep into
the inner recesses of Nickajack Cave near Chattanooga on the Tennessee
River. There in pitch darkness he met God and then miraculously was able

to crawl to the opening of the cave. There waiting for him was his future wife June Carter and his mother.[100] That was one of Cash's turning points, along with the birth of his son John Carter Cash, in getting serious about battling his addiction. Cash had relative freedom from drugs until attacked in 1981 by an ostrich that ripped his stomach open and broke several ribs. While in hospital, he became heavily re-addicted to painkillers. In 1983, his family and friends did an intervention, which included Cash's going to the Betty Ford Clinic. Cash commented: "I'm still absolutely convinced that the intervention was the hand of God working in my life, telling me that I still had a long way to go, a lot left to do. But first I had to humble myself before God."[101] Because of the enormous pain from sixteen failed jaw operations, Cash well understood the cunning, baffling, and powerful pull of self-medication.

In the midst of great trauma, Cash found that spiritual music helped bring him back from the despair of his addictions, saying:"Wherever I go, I can start singing one of them and immediately begin to feel peace settle over me as God's grace flows in. They're powerful, those songs. At times they've been my only way back, the only door out of the dark, bad places the black dog calls home." Cash began to find great strength in reading the bible and in prayer. He learned to stop hating himself, and to forgive himself and others, saying: "I've had my years in the wilderness...I had to finally accept it, you know, that God thought there was something worth saving, so who was I to say, 'You're wrong?' "[102]

During this time, Billy Graham became a personal friend and mentor. Billy Graham, said Cash, "was interested, but never judgmental...I've always been able to share my secrets and problems with Billy, and I've benefited greatly from his support and advice. He's never pressed me when I've been in trouble; he's waited for me to reveal myself, and then he's helped me as much as he can."[103] Johnny and June would eventually sing and share at almost three dozen Billy Graham Crusades in front of around two million people.

Many people do not know that he wrote a novel about the apostle Paul, saying: "If God could embrace an avowed and bloodthirsty enemy of his son Jesus Christ, he'd make a place for Johnny Cash."[104] Few were aware that he was an ordained minister, even performing weddings, including one for his daughter Kathy.[105]

Johnny Cash the pirate finished well. His last producer Rick Rubin drew out that which was best and truest about Johnny Cash, particularly in the video *Hurt*. Cash said: "Rick saw something in me that I didn't know was there anymore." Johnny Cash rediscovered what made him tick musically.[106]

Bono said that *Hurt* was perhaps the best video ever made.[107] Johnny Cash the ex-pirate commented:

> The Master of Life's been good to me…He gives me strength to face past illnesses, and victory in the face of defeat. He has given me life and joy where others saw oblivion.[108]

TITUS 1:7 *"not violent, not pursuing dishonest gain"*

What kind of self-respecting pirate isn't violent and doesn't pursue dishonest gain? We North Americans live in a culture that glorifies violence through many video games, movies, music and mixed martial arts. Our youth and young adults are being given hundreds of messages telling them that restraining one's anger or sexual attractions is uncool and unhealthy. Lurking behind our violence and anger is unresolved fear. Because fear makes us feel weak, we often convert our fear into aggression, making us feel in control. We men fear the feeling of helplessness. GK Chesterton noted that:

> most modern freedom is at root fear. It is not so much that we are too bold to endure rules; it is rather that we are too timid to endure responsibilities.[109]

Our glorification of violence makes us our own worst enemy. Our pride naturally leads to anger and aggression. Carter and Minirith hold that "loneliness creates anger." Loneliness is the empty feeling of isolation that leaves us on the outside looking in.[110] Pirates are naturally very lonely, angry people who trust no one. Only the Power from on High can radically change such people from the inside out into a new generation of healthy leaders.

It was said of Cretans, "They are so given to making gain in disgraceful and acquisitive ways that among the Cretans alone of all men, no gain is counted disgraceful."[111] The Cretans who were famous for their honey jars were said to "stick to money like bees to honey"![112] Through the power of the Holy Spirit, Paul was teaching Titus how to strengthen honest, generous ex-pirate leaders. Titus had earlier proved through his work with the Corinthians that he could be trusted with money, making him the perfect person to model financial faithfulness to the Cretans. That is why Paul said about Titus that "they were taking pains to do what is right, not only in the eyes of the Lord but also in the eyes of people."[113] Titus helped the Cretans move from being selfish takers to generous givers. Brian Kluth memorably commented: "Giving is saying to God "You are my source, you are my provider." Giving is the rubber that hits the road."[114]

A wise person once said to me: "If you want to know what is going on, follow the money". How people spend and receive money is a major clue to what they really value. False teaching usually has a financial reinforcement. False teachers are not usually false teachers for purely altruistic motives. Dishonest gain is all that pirates know as normal.

Many of us were raised with stories of hidden pirate gold buried on a deserted island. My late uncle Don Allen used to dive as a navy frogman for sunken treasure in the Caribbean. Treasure chests make me think about Long John Silver, the Swiss Family Robinson, Captain Kidd, and Treasure Island. It also reminds me of Jesus' parable for selling all for hidden treasure in a field.[115] It is so easy to lay up treasures foolishly for ourselves and not be rich towards God.[116] The Cretan ex-pirates would have learned from Titus that where their treasure was, there would be their heart also.[117] We ex-pirates have this amazing treasure in jars of clay.[118] But do we really value it? May this new generation of Tituses be healthy in how they handle their buried treasure.

When I was selected as the Rector of St. Simons NV, one of the wardens/elders told me that we are $10,000 behind from last year and if things do not turn around by June, we wouldn't be able to pay your salary. "No problem", I said, "God pays for what he orders." They felt better; I felt worse.

I met with our St. Simon's NV Church Council and just studied one biblical stewardship passage at each meeting. After a few months, one of the Church Council members said: "This is all very nice, Reverend, but when are we going to do something?" It seemed to me that we were doing something by educating our leaders first.

I had told our ladies group that they could no longer save the church with their garage sales. Rather they needed to give the money away to missions and outreach, an idea that caught on. Finally in June of that first year, I preached on the lectionary passage talking about tithing our first 10% and sacrificial giving above 10%. Some of our long-timers hit the roof. A medical specialist heard about the situation and began tithing that next Sunday. This action broke a log jam and released a flood of biblical generosity from which we have never looked back.

Every year at St. Simon's NV we have an annual Stewardship education time where we teach from the bible on biblical stewardship of our time, talent, and treasure, and where lay people share for two to three minutes why they tithe and give sacrificially. Each year before our annual Pledge Sunday, we have a twenty-four hour Stewardship Prayer Vigil. Financial stewardship and prayer are inseparably linked.[119] It is vital that we never ask anyone to do anything important that we do not ask them to first pray about, whether it is time, talent or treasure. As we seek the Lord in prayer about what we need to give, God speaks to us and softens our hearts. E. Stanley Jones said: "If I do not pray, I shall probably become cynical and shallow. If I do pray, I shall probably get nerve and courage, a sense of adequacy, power over wayward desires and passions."[120]

Biblical stewardship says no to arm-twisting, panic appeals or guilt. Our giving must be out of thanksgiving and love for what Jesus did on the cross. Our stewardship focus always wraps up with an annual pledge Sunday in mid-November where people bring in their pledge cards for the coming year.

For over eight years, I robbed God after becoming a Christian in 1972. By Anglican standards, I gave generously. While I believed in tithing, I was waiting until I felt financially secure enough to tithe. When I lost my voice in Dec 1980, I read Dr Peter Wagner's book "Your Spiritual Gifts can help your Church Grow" where he challenged people to tithe, saying that God would meet one's needs. Tithing is the only area in the bible where God says that we can put God to the test and see if he will not open the floodgates of heaven.[121] Everywhere else it is forbidden. As I had no income at the time, I figured that 10% of nothing was doable. God met my family's needs for the next 12 months, while I had a throat operation and then was able to go to St Matthew's Abbotsford as an assistant priest exactly 12 months after I had stepped down from St. Phillips Dunbar. Because God met my needs while I was out of work and couldn't speak, I figured that I couldn't stop tithing now that I had a job and income.

St. Simon's NV people have grown to realize that if they sow sparingly, they will reap sparingly (2 Corinthians 9:6). For the past twenty-five years, I have watched them sow generously and reap generously. I have seen God make all grace abound at St. Simon's NV so that having all they need, they have been able to abound in every good work. (2 Corinthians 9:10) St. Simon's NV used to be a mission congregation for many years, which meant it didn't pay its own way, and was almost closed several times by higher authorities. When St. Simon's NV started tithing, God enabled us to give partial support to missionaries around the world and locally. As AW Tozer put it, the best remedy for a sick church is to put it on a missionary diet.

When we were thrown out of our buildings after standing for the Lordship of Jesus Christ, God provided many financial miracles. We had a lot of startup costs in a new setting, and were in Dec 2005 down to five hundred dollars in the bank. There was a lot of pressure from a few people to drop our missionaries in order to balance the budget. But God spoke to me at the Anglican Mission Winter conference. I determined that I would not sacrifice our missionaries on the altar of meeting our budget. So we kept giving to our missionaries, and God miraculously came through. It is worth noting that the only time that the bible encourages us to be 'liberal' as Christians is financially, not doctrinally or morally.

God does not need your money. God is quite capable of looking after his bride without you. But God does love a cheerful, hilarious giver. Generosity is a healthy mark of a Spirit-filled ex-pirate. God is inviting you to model healthy leadership through being sacrificially generous in your local church and to missions.

TITUS 1:8 *"Love what is good"*

Goodness has a PR problem. Do you love what is good? While in Crete, I saw colourful boats everywhere, but instead of being used for piracy, they were dedicated to earning an honest living. God does not typically wipe our pre-Christian abilities but rather he redirects them to healthy, life-giving purposes. In such a way, we ex-pirates "provide for urgent needs and do not live unproductive lives." (Titus 3:14) CS Lewis once said that "No man knows how bad he is till he has tried very hard to be good."[122]

I remember being asked by a neighbour "What are you doing to do this New Year's Eve: Be good or party hard?" Being put on the spot, I paused and smiled, saying "I'm going to have to ask my wife." Later I thought, "Being good sounds rather boring to many people. Goodness almost needs a press agent to convince people of its value." Paul and Timothy were not trying to convince Cretan pirates to be "goody-goodies" or interfering "do-gooders", but rather through the power of the Holy Spirit to embrace the radical good that transforms a whole society. Life's most persistent and urgent question, said Martin Luther King Jr, is: "What are you doing for others?"[123] We are to overcome evil with good. Why are we here on earth? The Good Book says that we were created to do good works.[124] Bishop Sandy Millar memorably said: "Satan's attack is always the same: "You're no good, you never were any good, and you never will be any good."[125] The accuser tries to trap us in shame and guilt. Titus' impact on pirate leaders shows that goodness is not beyond anyone's reach.

What use is the good if we do not love it? How can we ever resist evil unless we hate the destructiveness of evil?[126] There are 655 verses on goodness in the Bible, 218 alone in the New Testament. In Titus, 22% of all the verses focus on doing goodness. In no other epistle, even in James, is there such an intensive and extensive emphasis on good works, seven times in just 46 verses. [127]

The eighteenth century liberal theologian Friedrich Schleiermacher rejected the authenticity of Titus, in part because of its emphasis on good works. But was the book of Titus teaching salvation by works? Hardly. Titus proclaims the shocking truth that even pirates can change. As Titus 3:5 clearly says, he saved us, not because of righteous things we had done, but because of his mercy. Paul was not teaching salvation by our own human effort. He was not telling us to pull us up by our own bootstraps. Rather Paul was teaching that good works are the natural fruit of the root of genuine faith in Jesus Christ. As CS Lewis put it, "the Christian does not think God will love us because we are good, but that God will make us good because He loves us." The Cretans as ex-pirates were radically committed to being healthy leaders where instead of being takers, they would be givers.

Some people mistakenly see the sixteenth century Reformation as an anti-good works movement. Martin Luther however taught that "good works do not make a good man, but a good man does good works."[128] It is not enough to just talk about goodness. Healthy leaders demonstrate practical goodness on a costly daily basis. That is why John Wesley memorably said:

> Do all the good you can, By all the means you can, In all the ways you can, In all the places you can, At all the times you can, To all the people you can, As long as ever you can.[129]

William Wilberforce as a healthy leader did lasting good by collaborating with John Newton, a former 'pirate' slave trader. Motherless at age six and sent to sea on his eleventh birthday, Newton soon became a teenage rebel. He was press-ganged into the Navy and flogged for desertion. Newton tragically became involved with the African Slave Trade. You name the corruption. He both saw it and lived it during his wealthy slave trading days. He even ended up for a short time as a slave himself. What he was most enslaved to, however, was a violent temper and a filthy tongue. Newton was so blasphemous that once even his hardened shipmates threatened to throw him overboard in order to calm a dangerous storm.

Throughout his blasphemy and rebellion, John had family members who never stopped praying for him. Secretly he began to read the Bible but somehow it never made sense. One night in March 1748, at the age of 23, he was on board a cargo ship which was fighting for its life against heavy seas and rough weather. Worn out with pumping and almost frozen, he called out for God's mercy at the height of the storm, and was amazed to be saved from almost certain death.

Newton's life had many twists and turns. Eventually he renounced his involvement with slave trading, and, at age 39, became an Anglican Priest. He persuaded the young William Wilberforce to stay in politics, and joined him in his fight to abolish the slave trade. After 40 years of prayer and hard work, Wilberforce, through Newton's influence, finally had slavery abolished in 1833, resulting in the liberation of over 800,000 Caribbean slaves on July 31st 1834.[130]

John Newton turned from death to life, from toxicity to health, from piracy to good. He celebrated his new life in Christ by writing one of the world's most famous songs:

> "Amazing Grace, how sweet the sound
> That saved a wretch like me.
> I once was lost but now am found,
> Was blind but now I see."

Sadly there are still today twenty-seven million people trapped in slavery and human trafficking. May the healthy leadership of Newton and Wilberforce cause us as North Americans to make a lasting global difference through loving the good.

Loving the good gives us the courage to face the bad and the unhealthy in our own lives. The key to becoming holistically healthy is by first admitting as the Book of Common Prayer puts it, that "there is no health in us." So many of us as leaders never get serious about our health until our GP tells us the bad news about our weight, our cholesterol, and our blood pressure. We won't necessarily listen to our spouse, our parents and our friends, but sometimes our GP can get our attention. I was struck by a poster at a local health food store that said: "Have you been eating badly and avoiding the gym? Stop saying 'I should' and say 'I will!'" Healthy leaders stop believing their unhealthy excuses.

At one of the gyms that I work out at, there are many senior citizens. Getting to know them, I have asked many why they work out. Invariably they tell me that it was after their stroke or their heart attack that their GP got them to the gym. A little voice in me keeps saying: "Why wait for a stroke or heart attack before we embrace a healthy lifestyle?" I need to model as a leader the healthy lifestyle that I am advocating for this new generation of healthy leaders. This can't be about 'do what I say, not what I do.' My being and doing must be convergently integrated if I am to finish well. This new generation of leaders has a very sensitive nose for hypocrisy.

In many parts of the world, the lack of food is their greatest problem. In North America, our greatest problem is too much food, resulting in high cholesterol, high blood pressure, hip, knee and back problems, and even cancer. Food is literally killing us as North Americans. Food, a good gift from God, has sadly become Public Enemy #1 in North America. And time is running out for many of us to turn this one around.

Growing waiting-lists for needed surgeries remind us of the crisis in our current health system. One doctor summarized the essence of modern medicine as either removing something (surgery) or putting something in (medication). All of us want to be holistically healthy. But do we want to be healthy badly enough to radically change our lifestyles? Are we willing to give up junk food, stop smoking, and start heading to the gym on a regular basis?

I remember having lunch with another man who told me that, in contrast to women, being overweight looked good on men. Perhaps this kind of rationalization explains why men are almost twice as likely to have a weight problem as women. Male clergy often suffer from the pastoral paunch, the fruit of too many congregants showing us love through food. Our most respectable sin, gluttony, is killing and crippling far too many North American leaders. It is a lie that we can eat whatever we want without tragic consequences. Pushing ourselves away from the table can be a radical act of biblical stewardship, of caring for our bodies as temples of the Holy Spirit.

When a leader makes the effort to be healthy in body, mind and spirit, it releases hope and faith in others. One of my favorite workout machines is the stationary bike. I enjoy it because it produces a good warm-up and also allows me to read without crashing! I enjoy doing Morning Prayer on the stationary bike. Silently reading the Book of Common Prayer not only makes the workout go much quicker, but also brings my spirit more alive. I had no idea years ago how health-conscious the Prayer Book is, as it speaks of "the healthful Spirit of Thy Grace" and "Thy saving health to all nations."[131] The Prayer Book has shown me that both in the physical and the spiritual, we can "dissemble and cloke" our laziness and "follow too much the devices and desires of our own hearts"[132]. Perhaps that is why "workouts in the gymnasium are useful, but a disciplined life in God is far more so, making you fit both today and forever." (1 Timothy 4:4 Message Translation) It's time to say no to being a spiritual and physical couch-potato! May each of us as ex-pirates show leadership by getting up off our couches and begin a healthy workout of our bodies, minds, and spirits.

TITUS 1:9 *"He must hold firmly to the trustworthy message as it has been taught, so that he can encourage others by sound doctrine and refute those who oppose it."*

We live in an age in which many people do not know what to hold firmly to anymore. Once violated, it is hard to restore trust. So many authority figures, including much of the institutional church, have let us down. So many North American women find it very challenging to trust and respect their husbands. It was not easy for Cretans, given their pirate heritage, to trust anyone. That is why Paul showed Timothy how to raise up unusually trustworthy leaders with an unusually trustworthy message. Without trust, community is impossible. Without trust, relationship dies. Without trust, our marriages and families end up in the wastebasket of postmodern cynicism.

Paul taught Titus' neophyte Cretan leaders about trustworthy leadership. The problem is always leadership. The solution is also leadership: godly leadership, healthy leadership submitted to the authority of Holy Scripture, leadership that takes seriously the Creed and the Thirty Nine articles, leadership that does not treat the Ten Commandments as multiple-choice. As Bishop John Rodgers put it, when the Church is sound, there is a great love in the heart of the Church for Scripture.[133] Theology and ethics are deeply integrated in Titus. Titus as a healthy leader did not just talk the talk; he walked the walk.

We all need encouragement to be healthy. Paul knew that the best way for Titus to strengthen the Cretans was through sound, healthy teaching. The Hebrew equivalent for the Greek word for health (hygiaino) is the term *shalom*.[134] As baby Christians, the Cretan ex-pirates desperately needed to be strengthened and discipled in the way of Christ. The less popular part of healthy discipling is saying no to false teaching. Our basic doctrine needs to be healthy and true, or everything goes toxic. That is why John Calvin said that "a pastor needs two voices, one for gathering the sheep and the other for driving away wolves and thieves."[135] False teaching by theological pirates is not to be benignly winked at. Without saying no to the false, we will never be transformed by the true. Without rejecting evil, we will never fully embrace the good. Goodness is actually good for you, healthy for you, life-giving for you. Evil is toxic and soul-destroying. May this new generation of healthy North American leaders have the transformational ability to say yes to the good and no to evil.

"What a gracious man", I thought as Dr J.I. Packer spoke. In the midst of a raging North Carolina snowstorm, he was giving a morning devotion at the *Anglican Mission* Winter Conference on John 21, in which he identified with Simon Peter's growing through failure.[136] The first time I ever spent time with Dr Packer was in 1979 in a student residence where we literally chased noises in the heating system. Dr Packer came across so humbly and natural, despite his worldwide reputation.

Dr J.I. Packer honoured me by writing the forewords to both my last book on 1 and 2 Timothy, and on this book on Titus. As a faithful teacher, Dr Packer holds firmly to the trustworthy message with grace and perseverance. Some believe that "J.I. Packer will be remembered as the principal theologian of the 21st Century."[137]

Healthy theology produces healthy leaders. Dr Packer teaches locally at Regent College in Vancouver. As such, we have been unusually privileged to have a new generation of students (including my middle son Mark) learn directly from Dr Packer's years of experience and wisdom. Recognized by Time Magazine as one of the twenty-five most influential evangelicals, Dr Packer is best known for his best-selling book *Knowing God*. In reading Dr Packer's doctoral thesis, I discovered that the heart of Dr Packer's vision is the evangelical renewal embodied in the wisdom of Richard Baxter. Baxter taught that knowing God is the very heart of salvation, that knowledge of God is what humans lost through the Fall and what is restored through Christ.[138] From Baxter, Dr Packer learned that "clergy are called to be physicians of the soul, prescribing for spiritual health of the soul."[139]

Richard Baxter wrote 168 books, many after the infamous 1662 ejection of Baxter and 2,000 other Anglican clergy from their pulpits.[140] Baxter held that he is not "the best scholar who hath the readiest passage from the ear to the brain, but he is the best Christian who hath the readiest passage from the brain to the heart."[141] This integration of heart and head in knowing God is a strong emphasis by Dr J.I. Packer as he warns against "hardness of heart and cynicism of the head."[142] Baxter was fearless in his stand against the slave trade, saying:

> To go as pirates and catch up poor negroes or people of another land, that never forfeited life or liberty, and to make them slaves, and sell them, is one of the worse kinds of thievery in the world.[143]

Baxter, like Titus, set people free from piracy. Even though Baxter's books were largely forgotten after the Great Eviction of 1662, they were later rediscovered by Philip Spener, the founder of European Pietism, by John Wesley who reintroduced Baxter to the English-speaking world, by William Wilberforce who was inspired to end the slave trade, by Charles Spurgeon, and most recently by Dr. JI Packer.[144] The title of CS Lewis' best-selling book *Mere Christianity* is taken directly from Richard Baxter.[145] This rediscovery of the practical, balanced wisdom of Richard Baxter and J.I. Packer is a key way forward for leaders who have lost their way in our post-modern, pirate culture. If the Cretans can be delivered from piracy through Titus, there is hope for even North Americans.

TITUS 1:10 *"For there are many rebellious people, mere talkers and deceivers..."*

Restoring health requires the unmasking of toxic deceptions. It was fascinating for me to visit the birthplace of the original Labyrinth movement, the Cretan palace of Knossos. In North America, due to the influence of new-age leader Dr Jean Houston and Lauren Artress from San Francisco's Grace Cathedral, labyrinths have been appearing everywhere, including at my old alma mater and the church where my grandmother had her funeral.[146] Ironically, the emphasis in the actual written documentation about Labyrinth usage was not **how to enter** the labyrinth but **how to escape** the labyrinth.

The labryinth story starts with King Minos, the legendary founder of the Cretan Minoan civilization. Minos rejected a beautiful bull offered him by a Greek deity. Because of this rejection, the Greek deity had Minos' wife have physical intimacy with another bull, giving birth to a troublesome son, the Minotaur, half bull/half human. To contain this difficult 'teenager', Daedalus built the labryinth, which essentially functioned as a prison for King Minos' awkward step-child.[147]

You all understand how hungry 'teens' can be. So King Minos demanded six young Athenian men and six young Athenian women to be sacrificed at the Labryinth where they would be eaten by his Minotaur step-son.

The book *Heritage Walks in Athens* comments that "in myth again, Athens' most important King was Theseus, son of Aigeus, who defeated the Minotaur and released the city from the vassal's tax paid to Crete."[148] Theseus escaped from the labyrinth after his girlfriend Princess Ariadne gave him the thread to follow out of the Labyrinth back to freedom.[149]

The term Labyrinth comes from the Lydian term *Labyrs* which means "double-headed ax", an object of cult worship among the Minoan Cretans.[150] While at the National Museum of Crete, I took a picture of an actual historic "Labyrs/Double-Edged Ax", an object of worship used in the labyrinth to devour the young.[151] The Labyrinth is the place of the sacred ax used ritually to decapitate victims while offering them to the sacred Minotaur bull. Similarly to the Canaanite/Philistine bull god Baal, the Cretan sacred bull was worshipped for its male sexuality and power.[152] Does the labyrinth have the capacity to "decapitate" the mind, bypassing our God-given ability to order our thoughts and think critically?

An ex-new-ager who attended our congregation participated a while back in the Labyrinth. Upon walking to the centre of the circle, she immediately sensed a dark spiritual vortex sucking her down.[153] Fortunately, being a Spirit-filled Christian, she later renounced her involvement in the Labyrinth and through prayer was cut free from the bondage that she was sensing.

Being westerners, we often fail to realize that seemingly harmless 'physical' techniques can have significant questionable spiritual impact on our lives.

An example of this might be how many people innocently get hooked into Hatha yoga through the guise of a community centre yoga course. Because Hatha yoga appears to westerners to be merely physical in nature, we fail to see the religious syncretism that we are involving ourselves in. Nothing from a Hindu perspective is merely physical, because for Hinduism, the physical is merely an illusion. So-called physical yoga asanas are designed to open the psychic door to the Hindu deities through ritual reenactment of specific Hindu deities. Community-Centre Yoga is in reality the 'marijuana' entry-level drug of the new age world.[154]

One of the patterns with the dozens of new-age fads sweeping North America and the West Coast in particular is that they all pop up out of the blue but claim to have rediscovered an ancient secret technique that we all need. Many of them, including the fast-growing Labyrinth fad, even reconstruct a plausible but misleading Christian history used to persuade well-meaning Christians.[155] The Labyrinth, as currently practiced, has very little to do with the Chartres Cathedral, and very much to do with Dr. Jean Houston's impact on the new-age-friendly Grace Cathedral in San Francisco.[156] The alleged Chartres connection is somewhat like a post-modern sound bite, a recently invented media-driven 'history'. There is no written history of labyrinth walking at Chartres. All we have is the fact of an unused labyrinth on the floor of the Chartres Cathedral. It is like an empty crab shell into which anything can crawl. Nature hates a vacuum. Is the Chartres situation being used as a legitimization for introducing new age practices into unsuspecting churches? There are also astrological symbols in the stained glass window at Chartres, but no one yet is recommending taking part in 'christian' astrology classes because of Chartres.

Dr. Jean Houston, who is ground zero for the labyrinth movement, was listed on the Internet as one of the 10 top New Age speakers in North America.[157] The inside cover of Jean Houston's 1997 book *A Passion for the Possible* describes herself as "considered by many to be one of the world's greatest teachers..." Of concern to renewal-oriented Christians is that

Houston teaches her students on the "Mystery School" how to speak in occult glossolalia. She encourages her participants to "begin describing your impressions in glossolalia" and even to "…write a poem in glossolalia."[158] This counterfeit phenomenon, of course, does not discredit the genuine Christian gift of tongues/glossolalia that is available after renouncing the occult, receiving Jesus as Lord, and asking for the filling of the Holy Spirit.

As a past president of the Association for Humanistic Psychology, Jean makes use of her doctorate in "Philosophy of Religion" to gain access to areas where most new-agers cannot go.[159] For example, as noted widely in media, she became a consultant to Hillary Clinton, helping her to 'channel' the spirit of Eleanor Roosevelt.[160]

The Labyrinth, also called the Dromenon[161], is the official symbol of Dr. Jean Houston's new-age 'Mystery School'.[162] Houston describes her Mystery School students as "…the dancers of the Dromenon…"[163] In Houston's 1996 book *The Mythic Life*, she credits H.F. Heard's novel *Dromenon* with its "psychophysical state of ecstasy and spiritual awakening" as the inspiration to adopting the image of the Dromenon/Labyrinth as the symbol of her work.[164] Heard, a Vedanta Yoga devotee of Swami Prabhavananda, was an early pioneer of the New Age and even the Hippy movements with his recommendation of LSD and fire walking as spiritual initiation exercises.[165] Jean Houston notes:

> Again I owe a considerable debt to Gerald Heard, for it was under the name of H.F. Heard that he published a remarkable fictional story 'Dromenon', the inspiration of which provided me with the naming of my own first center. In the story, an archeologist encounters a therapy in stone, a mystical transformation of body, mind and spirit…An example of the Dromenon can be found on page 1 (of Heard's book *The Great Fog*). This is the famous dromenon found on the floor of Chartres Cathedral. I often use this in my seminars by inscribing it on the floor and having the participants walk its pathways, always to great effect.[166]

Heard's novel tells the story of an architectural student who, with the help of an Orphic/hermetic soul-guide, gains gnostic enlightenment after dancing through a labyrinth concealed beneath a British church building.[167] The labyrinth dance, according to Heard, is meant to be a reenactment of the dancing Hindu deity Shiva, the definitive symbol of yoga.[168] Canon Lauren Artress from Grace Cathedral brought the Labyrinth back to her Cathedral after experiencing the Labyrinth at Jean Houston's Mystery School.[169] Artress notes that she was

> hardly prepared for the force of my own reaction. As soon as I set foot

into the labyrinth I was overcome with an almost violent anxiety. Some
part of me seemed to know that in this ancient and mysterious archetype,
I was encountering something that would change the course of my life.[170]

It is interesting that Artress, with her Cathedral connection, became far
more prominent in her labyrinth promotion than her new age mentor. Artress notes:

I worked with Jean Houston in her Mystery School in 1985. In 1986, I
was asked to serve as Canon Pastor at Grace Cathedral in San Francisco…
These programs eventually led me to the rediscovery of the labyrinth in
1991 when I returned to the Mystery School for one weekend.[171]

Jean Houston wrote in her book The Possible Human about "…the growth
of Dromenon (Labyrinth) communities."[172] As acknowledged in Labyrinth
websites, the Labyrinth is a mandala[173], which is actually a Hindu 'occult'
meditation process brought to the Western world by the grandfather of
the New Age, Dr. Carl Jung.[174] Is it a mere coincidence that the labyrinth
resembles the coiling of the yogic kundalini snake? Is the Labyrinth actually
a form of walking yoga? Might the labyrinth be a thinly disguised yogic
initiation rite into new age oneness, into the gnostic reconciliation of gender
opposites?[175] It is unthinkable for many westerners to imagine that walking
the labyrinth might yogically kill the mind and remove one's sense of self.

The Labyrinth has since spread to thousands of towns and cities. Artress
claimed that "over a million people have walked the labyrinth at Grace
Cathedral alone…"[176] Even the infamous Starhawk, the self-declared practicing witch and colleague of Matthew Fox, was reported to be walking
the labyrinth.[177] One of the stated purposes of the Labyrinth is to connect
us to the mother goddess, of which the labyrinth is a symbol. In her book
Walking A Sacred Path: Rediscovering the Labyrinth as a Spiritual Tool, Canon Artress states that "The labyrinth is a large, complex spiral circle which
is an ancient symbol for the divine mother, the God within, the goddess,
the holy in all creation."[178] Artress says that "You walk to the center of the
labyrinth and there at the center, you meet the Divine."[179] Jean Houston
claims that "As we encounter the archetypal world within us, a partnership
is formed whereby we grow as do the gods and goddesses within us."[180] To
Jean Houston, it seems that all of life is made up of polytheistic labyrinths.
In her book The Hero & the Goddess, she recommended: "Now, taking
a favorite god or goddess by the hand, a Greek one this time, explore the
labyrinthian winding of your left hemisphere…Take the deity by the hand
and begin to explore the labyrinth winding of your right hemisphere, the
place of intuition."[181]

It is also interesting how the current Dr Jean Houston-inspired Labryinth movement is so closely connected with the modern mother-god/dess revival movement. Dr. Jeffrey Satinover memorably comments that "Goddess worship" is not the cure for misogyny, but it is its precondition, whether overtly or unconsciously.[182] Goddesses as the productive deities were viewed as the most important in Cretan spirituality. In Cretan artwork, they were portrayed as the Queen of Wild Beasts, Kourotrophos (Nursing Mother of Youths), Mother and Daughter, the Goddess of the Serpents, and the Goddess of the Doves.[183]

Mother/father goddess worship is normative through most religions of the world. Consequently when the Judeo-Christian message of monotheism impacts a culture, mother-goddess worship is deeply affected. In Crete, the Lordship of Jesus Christ replaced the worship of male and female sexuality, of the mother/father goddess. It is not a neutral thing whom and what you worship. You become like what you worship. You act like that in which you really believe in. Your view of God is the highest truth about you, as it shapes everything you do. This is why the attempted reintroduction of mother/father goddess worship into many churches is of such significance.[184] As with Titus facing the Cretan Labryinth, a new generation of healthy leaders needs to be wise as serpents and harmless as doves.

Pirates by definition are rebellious deceivers. People liked to romanticize pirate ships, but in fact most were "damp, dark, cheerless places, reeking with the stench of bilge water and rotten meat."[185] Pirate ships suffered terribly from overcrowding and disease, with as many as 250 men crammed into a rat-infested ship just 127 feet long by 40 feet wide.[186] Our post-modern North American culture often resembles a stinking rebellious pirate ship, full of meaningless talk and deception. So many TV shows glorify violence, foolishness, and greed. Meaningless deception. Meaningless violence. Meaningless consumerism. Rebellion is the way of death. Godly health is the way of life.

This North American toxicity was foreshadowed in Titus 1:10-11 where false teachers were teaching things they ought not to teach. Have we not all sadly met church-goers whose "minds and consciences are corrupted. They claim to know God, but by their actions they deny him…?" Some may wonder what hope there is in such a time of theological and moral meltdown. Many North Americans have become stuck in despair. But there is a way forward in the wilderness. The answer to false teaching by false leaders is healthy teaching by healthy leaders.

TITUS 1:11 *"… They are ruining whole households by teaching things they ought not to teach, and that for the sake of dishonest gain."*

Household or home groups constituted the core of each church in the New Testament times. They still do two thousand years later. We need to do everything to strengthen and protect our home groups.[187] Paul is telling Titus that these wonderful home groups were being poisoned by false teachers who were financially preying upon the gullible. Dr. E Stanley Jones taught that 'the two greatest dangers to this emerging society, the Kingdom of God, come from two directions: money and power… Money and power crucified Jesus.[188].' Until money is put at the foot of the cross, until money becomes the servant and not the master, it will destroy all healthy relationships in our lives. E. Stanley Jones wisely wrote that "We will not be able to get complete victory in human living individually and collectively until we get it at the place of money."[189]

TITUS 1:12-13 *"One of Crete's own prophets has said it: 'Cretans are always liars, evil brutes, lazy gluttons.' This saying is true."*

Paul was quoting their own 6th Century B.C. prophet Epimenides, a native of Knossus near Heraklion, who lived about 600 BC. He was listed as one of the seven wise men of Greece.[190] Paul encouraged Titus to face how bad things were in Crete, not so that Titus would despair and leave, but so that Titus would stay and make a difference. Paul was passionate about life transformation of all people, even pirates. Paul knew that there are no sins too great for God to break through.

Dr William Barclay commented that "no people ever had a worse reputation than the Cretans. The ancient world spoke of the three most evil 'C's': the Cretans, the Cicilians, and the Cappadocians."[191] At the heart of any self-respecting pirate would be falsehood, violence and gluttony. According to Polybius the Greek historian,

> The Cretans, on account of their innate avarice, live in a perpetual state of private quarrel and public feud and civil strife…and you will hardly find anywhere characters more tricky and deceitful than those of Crete."[192]

Polybius goes on to say that there is no stigma attached, among the Cretans, to any manner of financial gain. On this pirate island, lying, violence and gluttony were normalized virtues. It was all that they had known for the past eight hundred years. George Orwell stated that in a time of universal deceit, telling the truth is a revolutionary act.[193] This is what Titus did in Crete. He started a truth revolution, a Jesus revolution through speaking truth to a pirate culture, not that dissimilar from our North American culture.

William Barclay commented that

> so notorious were the Cretans that the Greeks actually formed a verb 'kretizein', to cretize, which meant "to lie and to cheat"; and they had a proverbial phrase "kretizein pros Kreta" to cretize against a Cretan, which meant "to match lies with lies", as diamond cuts diamond.[194]

The ultimate con is to con a con. Cretans could lie with the best of them. Cicero the Roman statesman commented that even highway-robbery was seen as honorable by Cretans.[195] You can imagine what a stretch it would be for Cretans to worship a God who does not lie. Paul was alluding to Numbers 23:19 where it said clearly that God is not a man that he should lie. Lying is the way of death. Truth is the way of health and life.

We live in a culture that glorifies violence, whether mixed martial arts, hockey battles, or blood-spurting online video games. At the 2011 Vancouver Stanley Cup final, we saw what happens when drunk, angry fans turned destructive. Crete normalized such behaviour because all Cretans were pirates. The miracle was how the Holy Spirit radically transformed such a violent culture. North America is in desperate need of breaking its addiction to mindless violence. Violence is the way of death. Jesus is the way of life.

In the movie *Wall Street*, one of the anti-heroes played by Michael Douglas was promoting his new book "Greed is Good". We live in a culture that normalizes greed, consumerism, and selfishness. Francis Xavier insightfully commented:

> I have had many people resort to me for confession. The confession of every sin which I have known or ever heard of, and of sins so foul that I never dreamed of them, have been poured into my ear. But no person has ever confessed to me the sin of covetousness.[196]

Laziness can take many forms: physically lazy, emotionally lazy, mentally lazy, spiritually/morally/ethically lazy. Even workaholism can be a form of laziness, being too busy and lazy to redeem one's time, to say no to things that suck us dry. Benjamin Franklin memorably said in Poor Richard's Almanack 1739: "O Lazy Bones! Dost think God would have given thee arms and legs if he had not designed that thou should use them." He later said: "Up sluggard and waste not life; in the grave will be sleeping enough."[197] Laziness is often a symptom of our being paralyzed by our fears, our self-criticism, our feeling that we are inadequate and will never measure up.

Until Grade 10, I was always known as hard-working and conscientious at school. Once I decided that I was not going to be an engineer like my father, I became stuck and demotivated. I was lost and lacking direction. I had no idea who I was and what I was to do with my life. During my lost phase, I took an auto mechanics course in which I discovered how exhausting it was to be lazy and merely look busy. In the words of C.S. Lewis, laziness means more work in the long run.[198] Of the twenty-five people in the mechanics course, only two or three knew what they were doing. The rest of us leaned on the cars, looked into the engine, and tried to look busy. It was one of the most painful experiences that I remember in Grade 12. During this time of extreme boredom, John Edmondson, one of the people who actually understood cars, invited me to a home group that totally changed my life. My laziness, my stuckness, was transformed into a new dynamism, a new excitement, a new reason to live that deeply impacted our high school. In the next few months, we organized rock concerts, brought in speakers, and handed out our own self-produced pamphlets to hundreds of other lost young people in our local high school. Looking back, I am amazed at all that we young leaders accomplished in such a short time, largely because we did not know better. If we had known how hard it was supposed to be, our lazy side might never have started.

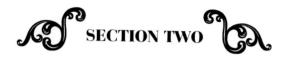

SECTION TWO

Strengthening the Generations

(Titus Chapter 2)

TITUS 2:1 *"You must teach what is according with sound/ healthy doctrine."*

Titus was commissioned by Paul to be a teacher of healthy faith and action. The pirate island of Crete was definitely not a healthy place when Titus arrived there. Paul identified different age and gender groups that Titus should teach in restoring health to Crete. The call to teach (didaskalia/didache) is used ten times in the forty-six short verses in Titus. Teaching others to teach others is at the heart of strengthening healthy leadership. Mature women were counterculturally taught by Titus to teach what is good. Doctrine (doctrina) is a Latin term for teaching. Without healthy doctrine, nothing changes. Teaching Cretan and North American pirates to become healthy is to be holistically done by both words and example.

One of the greatest teachers of healthy, sound living in the past one hundred years was Dr. E. Stanley Jones, a missionary for fifty years in India. Dr Jones said that: "the greatest source of power for physical health is the absence of inward clash and strife in the spirit."[199] Because God wills health in body, mind and spirit, we need to co-operate with God's will in this area. As we learn to surrender our fears and worries to the Lord, we are co-operating with God's Kingdom will for our lives. Dr Jones wisely commented that we have to trust to rest.[200] Letting go and letting God is at the heart of a healthy lifestyle. Only then can perfect love cast our all fear. Fear cripples our lives, our health, our communities. Pirates for all their bravado are very fearful, anxious people. Only the power of the Holy Spirit can set North American pirates free from the strongholds of fear and worry.

TITUS 2:2 *"Teach the older men to be temperate, worthy of respect, self-controlled, and sound in faith, in love and in endurance."*

We all know the expression: "You can't teach an old dog new tricks." Yet Titus was expected to teach old sea dogs how to be healthy. The older men in Crete were lifelong hardened pirates. To be temperate, respectable, self-controlled and healthy was not on their radar screen. Yet it was exactly what was needed for the transformation of this pirate island.

Thomas Lea comments that:

"the latter years of life, especially for men, can be filled with regrets, a sense of uselessness or worthlessness, feelings of despair, self-absorption, or even a tendency to relax moral standards because of old age."[201]

Dr Gil Stieglitz, commenting on the challenges of aging, said: "Life is one big loss. We all, like Job, lose everything in the end. We lose our youth, dreams, jobs, catastrophic loss, divorce, affairs, cancer."[202] Because men tend to be more isolated, it is often harder for men to cope with these painful losses.

Paul did not want older men to live grumpy, defeated lives, but rather to see themselves as missionaries to a pirate culture. Maturity is about investing in a new generation of healthy leaders. So many baby boomers still think that it is all about them. Dr Terry Walling said that baby boomers may be the most selfish generation in history. It does not need to end that way. Dr Michael Griffiths comments that many older men will face the temptation of being:

sour and cynical, self-centered and unloving. Losing the bright expectancy of youth, they become hard and brittle and resent every inconvenience. Thus they need to become 'sound in faith, in love and in endurance'[203]

Commenting on the movie 'Grumpy Old Men', Patrick Arbore said that:

many older men he counsels are angry all the time. It's as if anger is the only emotion they are able to express. What happens to older men is that they retreat into isolation. Men retreat into themselves, into their heads. There's this feeling of 'there's no escape.'[204]

Anger is our greatest challenge as men. Anger is a death wish. Unless we deal with our anger and frustration, we cripple our future. Too many men these days are crashing and burning, giving up on life and their potential to make a lasting difference in others. Angry men do not finish well. Frustration is so often a polite word for anger. I remember in a previous church when I was meeting with a man who told me that he was not angry; he was just frustrated. One day he came back to me and told me that he got it. His boss had said to him: "I'm frustrated", to which the man said: "Oh, you're angry". "No, I'm not!" said the boss. "I'm just ticked off!" The *Marriage Encounter* book mentions that the only two emotions traditionally allowed for men were anger and sex. Paul teaches Titus and the Cretan older men a better way to be healthy/sound in faith, love and endurance.

Dr Richard Campbell said to me that:

Of 400 male leaders in the Bible, only 80 finished well. All 80 would both take counsel and seek a rebuke. Five qualities that the 80 showed were intimacy with God, humility, faith, obedience, and the ability to take advice from others.[205]

There is no retirement in the bible, rather only being retreaded, renewed, restored for God's Great Commission and Great Commandment. The only retirement from serving in the bible is our being called home to glory. Since the 1930s, there has been a 440% increase in the number of North Americans over the age of 65, more than three times the population increase.[206] The ministry possibilities in reaching this burgeoning mission field are huge. Stuart Briscoe said:

> ...the older men have much to offer. They must not quit; they must not become self-absorbed; they must not become cranky and disgruntled. They must keep the faith and keep their cool and keep on keeping on.[207]

Dr Chuck Swindoll has wisely given up five tips for staying vital as we mature:

> Your mind is not old, keep developing it.
> Your humor is not over, keep enjoying it.
> Your strength is not gone, keep using it.
> Your opportunities have not vanished, keep pursuing them.
> God is not dead, keep seeking Him.[208]

It's never too late. My paternal grandparents had left Vancouver in 1959 to becoming a 'pioneering family' in an area of Roberts Creek that didn't even having running water or electricity. Grandpa Vic Hird, who was a 60-year-old master mechanic and second-generation blacksmith, decided to tent with his wife Olive while building their own house in the Roberts Creek woods. Each morning they trekked down to Flume Creek with the other pioneers to collect their daily water.

To help his parents build their house, my engineering father, accompanied by his young family, would take the Langdale Ferry many weekends to the Sunshine Coast. My strongest memory of the Sunshine Coast house-building spree was when I stepped on a long construction nail and had to be driven to my Grade One class for the first two months. My Grandfather worked so hard building his house and digging a well through 'hardpan' that he suffered a heart attack and promptly decided that he would be dying within a year. For the next 32 years of Grandpa's life on the Sunshine Coast, we 'knew' that Grandpa would be dead within about a year. Surprisingly all the healthy people died before Grandpa Hird.

Grandpa Vic sang in a church choir until he became an atheist when his first wife died. His deep love for children brought out the best in him. He had a soft spot for our eldest son James who was key to Grandpa coming back to faith in Jesus Christ. When James was about two to three years old, he danced before Grandpa Vic, as Grandpa Vic cathartically sang 'Jesus loves me, this I know for the Bible tells me so. Little ones to him belong, they are weak but he is strong. Yes, Jesus loves me, Yes Jesus loves me, Yes Jesus loves me. The Bible tells me so.' Grandpa Vic the atheist began listening to hymns again.

Later on Easter weekend, Grandpa Vic Hird surprised me again as he sang to me:

> Low in the grave He lay, Jesus my Savior,
> Waiting the coming day, Jesus my Lord!
> Up from the grave He arose,
> With a mighty triumph o'er His foes,
> He arose a Victor from the dark domain,
> And He lives forever, with His saints to reign.
> He arose! He arose!
> Hallelujah! Christ arose!

Grandpa Vic's spiritual breakthrough taught me that atheism is often a grief response to undealt-with trauma in one's life. Grandpa Vic did not know how to grieve, so he became stuck for several decades, until a little child led him back to the Lord. Grandpa got his song back. I had the privilege of sharing about this breakthrough when I took Grandpa Vic's funeral. There are many people in North America who have toxically lost their song. May a new generation of healthy leaders guide them back to their lost song.

When mature men become healthy in faith, love, and endurance, they become role models for a new generation of healthy leaders. They show that it is possible to get up again after being knocked down. It is possible to hold fast to the promises of God when everything is falling apart. This new generation of leaders is looking for healthy mentors and coaches who are finishing well, who are integrated in both their being and doing, their talking and walking. God is looking for you. Stop hiding in your pirate den.

TITUS 2:3 *"Likewise, teach the older women to be reverent in the way they live, not to be slanderers or addicted to much wine, but to teach what is good..."*

Many of the female pirates were addicted to gossip and alcohol. Paul challenged Titus to strengthen a new generation of healthy older women. This healthy new generation will talk directly to people rather than indirectly about them. This new generation will turn to Jesus in their pain rather than to self-medication.

While working out at a local gym, I met Mary Poppins (as her friends call her), the 85 year old lady who ran the Vancouver Sun Run and was put on TV. BJ McHugh did not start running until she was 55. Contrary to my guess, she was never a PE instructor, but rather a nurse. Recently she, with her son and granddaughter all ran the Honolulu Marathon. It's never too late for North Americans of any age to get healthy in body, mind and spirit. What are you waiting for?

TITUS 2:4 *"Then they can train the younger women to love their husbands and children..."*

This kind of love is not the agape love of laying your life down, but rather 'friendship' love (philandros). Older women are being challenged to teach younger women how to be the best friends of their husbands and children, to hang out with them and even play together. The purpose of this mentoring of younger women by older women is that no one would malign the word of God. When gossip and substance abuse are replaced with being the best friends of one's husband and children, God gets the glory.

Nana Allen, my maternal grandmother, was a truly amazing lady who mentored her daughter Lorna and others in the Christian faith. She was a devout Anglican Christian who loved the Book of Common Prayer, and knew that something was being tampered within the DNA of Anglicanism. Something healthy was becoming spiritually toxic. Nana knew that I would become an Anglican priest, and told me this, years before I even came to personal faith. I was convinced that I would become an electrical engineer like my father. Nana was very close to God and heard his still small voice. Her desire was to live until I became a deacon (which she did) and then to live until I became a priest (which she did). She died shortly before my throat operation on May 25th 1982 when God restored my voice. Nana was a healthy godly example of how older women can revolutionize their world for Christ.

TITUS 2:6-7 *"Similarly, encourage the young men to be self-controlled. In everything set them an example by doing what is good..."*

Paul knew that the greatest need of younger males was self-control. It is not a co-incidence that most people in prison are younger men under thirty. Male testerone can easily end up in destruction and chaos when not harnessed. Franklin D. Roosevelt said: "We cannot always build the future for our youth, but we can build our youth for the future." Masculinity is meant to be a force for good, for creation, not destruction. Transformed younger men are a powerful witness to the resurrected Christ. Titus as a younger man was not just to teach younger men, but also to demonstrate it in the way he lived. Paul's aim in verse eight is that Titus and these younger men would be so healthy that others would have nothing bad to say about them. People are watching everything we say and everything we do to see if we are genuinely healthy, authentically sound. AW Tozer said: "When unsaved people see your good works, you have taken away their weapons; you have taken their gun out of their hands."

Pirates and dictators always target angry young men. Dietrich Bonhoeffer, as a modern-day Titus, taught young men healthy self-control. Martyred for his faith just 23 days before the Allies liberated Germany, Bonhoeffer's last poem and his Barmen Declaration are printed in the 'Lutheran' hymnbook.[209]

Coming from a highly educated, aristocratic family, Bonhoeffer shocked his family by deciding to become a pastor.[210] Bonhoeffer was spiritually impacted by his Moravian Brethren 'nanny' Maria Horn who introduced him to the practice of having daily devotions.[211] After earning his doctorate at age 21, Bonhoeffer moved to the United States where he encountered African-American gospel music and preaching at the 14,000-member Abyssinian Baptist Church in Harlem, NY. The Abyssinian Church was led by Dr Adam Clayton Powell Sr, the son of slaves whose mother was a full-blooded

Cherokee. Dr Powell told a powerful story of his conversion to Christ from heavy drinking, violence and gambling.[212] Bonhoeffer was deeply moved by Dr Powell, saying "...here one can truly speak and hear about sin and grace and the love of God...the black Christ is preached with rapturous passion and vision."[213]

Moving back to Germany in 1931, Bonhoeffer warned people about the dangers of Nazism, but many brushed off his prophetic statements as alarmist. The Nazi Third Reich was a pirate empire. The Nazis worked carefully to first silence and then take over the Churches in Germany, birthing a movement called the German Christian Movement which discarded the Old Testament, putting the swastika at the centre of the cross.[214] At the Berlin Sports Stadium in 1933, in front of 20,000 supporters, the cross was denounced as 'a ridiculous debilitating remnant of Judaism, unacceptable to National Socialists.'[215] Nazis believed that it was un-aryan to let Jesus take our sins on the cross. They functioned as religious pirates, taking over churches and hoisting their own swastika flags.

Bonhoeffer responded by forming the Confessing Church movement which rejected racism and hatred of others. The Confessing Church started five seminaries/centres for training future young pastors. Many Confessing Churches were firebombed by gangs of Hitler Youth. On December 1935, the Nazis declared the Confessing Church to be illegal. They forbid the Confessing Church to hire employees, send out newsletters, take collections, or train students for ordination.[216] In 1937, the Nazis banned worship services from being held in unconsecrated buildings, homes or in public meeting halls. It also became illegal to pray for anyone who had been sent to prison.[217] Many Confessing Church pastors ended up in prison.

In 1938, Bonhoeffer quietly contacted Admiral Wilhelm Canaris who was involved in the German resistance movement. As the leader of the Abwehr Intelligence, Canaris was seeking for a way to remove Hitler.[218] After the annexation of Austria and the destruction of three hundred synagogues and 7500 Jewish-owned businesses on the night of Kristallnacht, Bonhoeffer was persuaded to return to the United States. His friends were sure that Hitler was about to destroy Bonhoeffer. He had no peace in the USA, knowing that Germany needed him. Bonhoeffer opened his bible to the verse: 'He who believes does not flee.' After only four weeks, he embraced his destiny, taking the last ship back to Germany.[219]

After the invasion of Poland and then France, Bonhoeffer was now required to report regularly to the police. He was forbidden to speak in public or publish books.[220] In 1943, while working for the underground, Bonhoeffer fell in love with and became engaged to Maria von Wedemeyer. Three months later he was arrested by the Gestapo. "Your life would have been quite different, easier, clearer, simpler, had not our paths crossed," he wrote to her. But Maria stayed faithful to Bonhoeffer to the very end.[221] While in Tegel Prison, Bonhoeffer wrote: "Church is only church when it is there for others." One of the guards, Sergeant Knobloch, tried to smuggle Bonhoeffer out disguised as a mechanic. But Bonhoeffer rejected the escape plan in order to protect his fiancée and family.[222] A British fellow prisoner said later that 'Bonhoeffer was all humility and sweetness with a deep gratitude for the mere fact that he was alive.'[223] After Bonhoeffer was hanged at Flossenburg, the prison doctor reported: "In the almost fifty years that I worked as a doctor, I have hardly ever seen a man die so entirely submissive to the will of God."[224] Bonhoeffer, as a modern day Titus, made a way forward for a new generation of healthy leaders.

TITUS 2:9 *"...to show that they can be fully trusted so that in every way they will make the teaching about God our Saviour attractive."*

Honesty is remarkably attractive and often very countercultural. More than 50% of the Greek population in Titus' day were slaves.[225] How would you like to have been the slave of Cretan pirates? This despised social class was very open to the transforming good news of Jesus Christ. Christianity was known as a slave religion. Christians often secretly worshipped in underground catacomb cemeteries. Ninety percent of the names engraved on the catacomb walls were slaves or ex-slaves.[226] Many slaves were well-educated, skilled prisoners of war or of piracy.[227] In ancient times the term 'slave' and 'thief' were interchangeable. In classical comedies, slaves were famous for mocking their masters.[228] Christlike slaves won their master's families for Christ by neither mocking nor stealing from their master. As all Cretans were lying pirates, the trustworthiness of their Christian slaves must have been very shocking, making the teaching about God our Saviour very attractive. In North America where dishonesty and unreliability are almost normal, is your yes 'yes' and your no 'no'? Can your boss trust you? Can other employees count on you, or are you all talk? Do you desire to be part of a new generation of healthy leaders that will transform this pirate continent?

I can imagine Titus agreeing with what Louis Pascal said in his book

Pensees: "Make religion attractive, make good men wish it were true, and then show that it is. Worthy of reverence because it really understands human nature. Attractive because it promises true good."[229] Are your friends, family and co-workers more attracted to Christ because of you? Do you as an ex-pirate make other North Americans wish that Christ is really true?

Many people naively say that religion is inherently bad. The Bible teaches in James 1:27 that there is genuine religion which cares for widows and orphans, and is not polluted by the world. Jesus is opposed to counterfeit religion, not the genuine. E. Stanley Jones commented: "We are all incurably religious. Even the communists, though repudiating religion, are deeply religious...Religion is a cry for life."[230] Religion is not the problem for North Americans. The real question is whether or not your religion is life-giving and relational. Does your religion make you more healthy or more toxic?

TITUS 2:11 *"For the grace of God that brings salvation has appeared to all people."*

The infamous Roman Emperor Nero was officially described as 'lord and saviour of the world'. Similarly Emperor Domitian required his subjects to call him Dominus et Deus noster, 'our Lord and God'.[231] Titus 2:13 radically states that Jesus, not Caesar, is our divine saviour. Jesus alone is Lord. Christmas even in our very secular culture still has a lot of appeal as the most celebrated holiday in North America. Islam affirms the virgin birth of the Messiah Jesus, while simultaneously denying his incarnation as our great God and Saviour in a manger.[232] Jesus' first appearing two thousand years ago taught Cretan pirates to say no to corruption and yes to godly healthiness. Only leaders who can say no have the ability to say yes. Unhealthy leaders either get stuck in negativity or naivety. Dr. E. Stanley Jones said that Christianity is cosmic optimism with scars on it.[233] Jesus' divine yes to us is stronger than any 'no' that might come from others or even ourselves.

Ex-pirate leaders live expectantly between two advents, Jesus' first and second coming. These two advents are described in Titus and Timothy as epiphanies, as breaking in of light into darkness.[234] The Cretan pirates' transformation was indeed from darkness to light. As Hank Williams sang, "I saw the Light. I saw the Light. No more in darkness. No more in night." Epiphanies brings leadership breakthrough. Healthy Christ-centered leaders are always passionate about the blessed hope of his glorious appearing, because they know that Jesus will return suddenly when least expected. Cretan pirates would have naturally been drawn to Jesus' describing his return as like a thief in the night. Healthy leaders know that time must be redeemed, not wasted because it is very short.

Islam affirms the second coming of Jesus while simultaneously denying Jesus' death and resurrection.[235] Paul said in 1 Corinthians 15:32 that if Jesus is not risen, let us eat, drink and be merry, for tomorrow we die. The Cretan pirates discovered through Titus that only the shed blood of Jesus on the cross could redeem them from all wickedness. Only Jesus' substitutionary sacrifice on the cross could purify rebellious pirates into becoming a peculiar people, a people who belonged to Jesus. Rather than Judas taking Jesus' place on the cross, Jesus took our place as a full, perfect and sufficient sacrifice, oblation and satisfaction for the sins of the whole world.[236] Only the finished work of Jesus on the cross can cause pirates to become eager to do what is good. The term 'peculiar people' alludes to the covenant language of Exodus 19:4-5 and 1 Peter 2:9 where God describes us as Kings and Cohens/Temple Leaders. The Cretan pirates went from being independent rebels to becoming a holy nation, a covenant family.[237]

Dr. Sam Shoemaker, co-founder of Alcoholics Anonymous, said that "the cross is a frontal attack of God upon man's pride. Its first and chief message is 'you cannot save yourself.'"[238] Cretan pirates were famous for their arrogance and pride. Our North American culture is often shamelessly loud and proud. We have forgotten that pride is the deadliest of the seven deadly sins. We North Americans are defiantly proud about being proud. The good news is that Jesus humbly gave himself on the cross for the proud and the arrogant. Gratitude for the cross brings the death of our North American pirate pride. Revival, renewal, and healing comes when we lay our pirate chests on the foot of the cross. Henry Blackaby, author of *Experiencing God,* said that revival is blocked by unconfessed sin in our lives: "The forgiveness of sin is the condition for the healing of our land."[239] Proud North Americans have little awareness how desperately that we need God's forgiveness.

TITUS 2:15 *"These, then, are the things you should teach. Encourage and rebuke with all authority. Do not let anyone despise you."*

This verse reminds me of Paul's saying in 1 Timothy 4:12: "Do not let anyone look down on you because you are young…" Do not let these pirates treat you with contempt, belittle you, and undermine you. Do not be afraid not only to encourage but also when necessary to rebuke and challenge. Be a fearless teacher rather than a people pleaser. Do not give up self to people who want to project their anxiety onto you. Sabotage and pushback will happen. Stay calm, stay focused, stay Christ-centered. Be a non-anxious catalyst. Embrace your full humanity in Christ. When Titus chose to be himself in Christ, he strengthened a new generation of healthy leaders. And so can you.

I knew of a pastor who occasionally fell into people-pleasing, letting himself be manipulated. Once he was so hurt that for a couple hours, he was done. A clergy friend said to him: "Have you prayed about it? (no) Have you consulted with other leaders? (no) This doesn't sound like you." At that point, he woke up from his downward spiral, and chose to be a Titus. Do not let anyone despise you. Don't let the pirates take you out. My life verse is 1 Corinthians 15:58: "Stand firm. Let nothing move you. Always give yourselves fully to the work of the Lord because your labour in the Lord is never in vain."

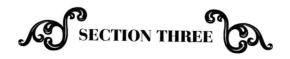

SECTION THREE

Strengthening Other's Health

(Titus Chapter 3)

TITUS 3:1 *"Remind the people to be subject to rulers and authorities, to be obedient, to be ready to do whatever is good"*

How ready are we independent North Americans to obey anyone? Pirates are normally the last people to be accountable to rulers and authorities. Captain Jack Sparrow's response to authorities was to swing on a rope towards the nearest pirate ship. Polybius, the Greek historian, said that Cretans were constantly involved in insurrections, murders, and internecine wars.[240] How in the world did this new accountability happen in Crete? How did they become ready to do whatever is good? Only the gospel could do this miracle. John Calvin said: "By nature, we all want power, and so no one wants to submit to anyone else."[241] If Cretans can become accountable, then North Americans have no excuse.

TITUS 3:2 *"…to slander no one, to be peaceable, and considerate, and to show true humility towards all people."*

Dr John Stott said that there are:

> in the end only two possible responses to the Word of God. One is to humble ourselves and tremble at it. The other is harden our hearts, stiffen our necks, and reject it.[242]

Jesus said: "Blessed are the peacemakers for they shall be called children of God." Peacemakers choose to take the lower seat. It is not easy for either powerful pirates or politicians to be humble peacemakers. This is a miracle of the Holy Spirit. One notable peacemaker was President John Adams. His greatest strength and weakness was that he was a humble peace-maker, even at the cost of sabotaging his own re-election as the second American President. In 1797, Napoleon captured 300 American ships. The 'hawks' in Adams' own Federalist party desperately wanted to go to war with France, but Adams negotiated a peace treaty that allowed him to disband Hamilton's unnecessary and costly army. Hamilton, the commander of this army, took this as a personal insult, and dedicated himself to splitting Adams' own Federalist Party.

With two Federalist presidential candidates, the Republican presidential candidate, Thomas Jefferson, won the election on the 37th ballot after a deadlocked tie vote. Jefferson, who had foolishly endorsed the blood-thirsty French Revolution, was wisely mentored by Adams. At his final State of Union address, President Adams stated: "Here and throughout our country, may simple measures, pure morals, and true religion, flourish forever!" It is too easy to cynically dismiss the possibility of pure morals for public leaders. Titus 1:15 incisively says: "To the pure, all things are pure, but to those who are corrupted and do not believe, nothing is pure." Adams' final prayer as he left the House was: "I pray Heaven to bestow the best of Blessings on this House and all that shall hereafter inhabit it. May none but honest and wise Men ever rule under this roof." Despite strong political differences, Adams and Jefferson ended as good pen pal friends, both dying on the significant American July 4th holiday.

As a healthy leader, John Adams was both passionate about liberty and yet cautious about our human tendency to selfishness. James Grant commended Adams for "his unqualified love of liberty, and his unsentimental perception of the human condition." As such, Adams produced constitutional boundaries that guarded sinful people's essential freedoms of life and liberty of speech, assembly, and religion. The US Congress praised Adams for his "patriotism, perseverance, integrity and diligence." Adams insightfully commented: "our Constitution was made only for a moral & religious people. It is wholly inadequate to the government of any other."

Adams has been described as one of North America's greatest bibliophiles. Healthy leaders are lifelong learners. Adams read voraciously in wide-ranging areas of interest, including the Bible. Equality for Adams was grounded in equal access to education for all: "knowledge monopolized, or in the Possession of a few, is a Curse to Mankind. We should dispense it among all Ranks. We should educate our children. Equality should be preserved in knowledge." His prayer for his children was: ""Let them revere nothing but religion, morality, and liberty."

One of Adams' leadership strengths was that he was deeply honest, even to his own political detriment. Unlike the worldly-wise Benjamin Franklin, he would say exactly what was on his mind. Adams urged Franklin to get more exercise, saying that "the sixth Commandment forbids a man to kill himself as it does to kill his neighbour. A sedentary life is tantamount to suicide." James Grant commented that "like the mythical George Washington, he seemed incapable of telling a lie; he was naturally and organically honest." Adams once commented: "The Ten Commandments and the Sermon on the Mount contain my religion." Adams the peacemaker was indeed an unusual politician. He found the endless political bickering to be painful and pointless, commenting that "a resolution that two plus two makes five would require fully two days of debate." Adams was known as a foul-weather politician, only drawn to serve his country because of the intense crisis. He would have much rather been anywhere else. Healthy leaders often make deep sacrifices for the sake of others. Adams was a latecomer to American Independence, preferring to work for peaceful reconciliation with the British. Because of his endless negotiations in France, Holland and England, Adams only saw his dear wife for a grand total of three months over six years. "Happy is the man who has nothing to do with politics and strife.", Adams wrote to Josiah Quincy on Oct 6th 1775.

Like Titus, Adams knew that healthy leadership must be rooted in prayer. One of Adams' first assignments in Congress was to draft a resolution appointing a day of fasting, humiliation, and prayer throughout the thirteen colonies: "that we may, with united hearts and voices, unfeignedly confess and deplore our many sins, and offer up our joint supplications to the all-wise Omnipotent, and merciful Disposer of all events; humbly beseeching him to forgive our iniquities, to remove our present calamities, to avert those desolating judgments with which we are threatened, and to bless our rightful sovereign, King George the third." Sadly King George dismissed Adams and his colleagues as 'wicked and desperate persons.' It is far too easy to label our opponents as pirates rather than humbly seek peaceful reconciliation.

King George's thirty-three thousand British troops resulted in thirty-five thousand American deaths by sword, sickness, or captivity. Adams knew that without heart-forgiveness, American independence would quickly become as barbaric as the French Revolution: "In a time of war, one may see the necessity and utility of the divine prohibitions of revenge and the Injunctions of forgiveness of Injuries and love of Enemies, which we find in Christian Religion. Unrestrained, in some degree by these benevolent Laws, Men would be Devils, at such a Time as such." Healthy leaders are humble forgivers.

In 1815 he wrote his own gravestone epitaph: "Here lies John Adams, who took upon himself the responsibility of the peace with France in the year 1800." May God strengthen a new generation of healthy North American peace-makers like President John Adams.

TITUS 3:3 *"At one time we too were foolish, disobedient, deceived and enslaved by all kinds of passions and pleasures. We lived in malice and envy, being hated and hating one another."*

We only have one choice: the foolishness of hatred or the wisdom of love. It is so easy to self-righteously think that we are better than others. Our hearts, said Jeremiah 19:9, are deceitful and desperately wicked. Who can understand them? Cretan pirates were famous for being hated and hating one another. Hatred is the way of death. Martin Luther King Jr. notably said that "hatred paralyzes life; love releases it. Hatred confuses life; love harmonizes it. Hatred darkens life; love illumines it." Piracy is all about the love of sex, money and power, putting them above God's Kingdom. Through Titus' healthy leadership on Crete, the love of power was replaced by the power of love. The late Marilyn Monroe confessed: "I always felt insecure and in the way, but most of all I felt scared. I guess I wanted love more than anything else in the world." Even North American pirates need love.

TITUS 3:4 *"But after that the kindness and love of God our Saviour toward man appeared..."*

In the midst of our foolishness, our disobedience, our malice and envy, Jesus the divine Saviour turned up and set us free. Only the kindness and philanthropic love of Jesus can bring about such a miracle. We suffer from a love deficit. Our biggest problem, said the late Ray Stedman, is our lack of love, our inability to love one another. Jesus is love incarnate. One of the most well-known children's songs throughout the world is "Jesus loves me, this I know." Somehow that song, like "Amazing Grace", forms part of the spiritual memory banks of most adults.

As a teenager, I found church boring and avoided it by golfing and skiing on Sunday mornings. But as a child, I remember enjoying Sunday School and looking forward to going. I've always liked to sing, and one of my favorite hymns as a child was "Jesus loves me, this I know". Even though I did not know Jesus personally, something touched me as I sang that song in Sunday School. Years later, I still feel deeply moved by this simple song.

Dr. Karl Barth was one of the most brilliant and complex intellectuals of the twentieth century. He wrote volume after massive volume on the meaning of life and faith. A reporter once asked Dr. Barth if he could summarize what he had said in all those volumes. Dr. Barth thought for a moment and then said: "Jesus loves me, this I know, for the Bible tells me so."

When Mao Tse Tung attempted to crush the church in China, things seemed very bleak. In 1972 however, a message leaked out which simply said: "The 'this I know' people are well". The Communist authorities did not understand the message. But Christians all around the world knew instantly that this referred to the world's most famous children's hymn. Miraculously the Chinese Church, instead of being crushed, has boomed under persecution, growing from 1.5 million believers to over 140 million.

The author of this amazing little children's song was Anna Bartlett Warner, sister to the famous 19th century writer, Susan B. Warner. Susan's first novel *The Wide Wide World* was an instant success, second only to *Uncle Tom's Cabin*, the most popular 19th century novel written in North America. Anna published her own novel *Dollars and Cents* under the pseudonym "Amy Lothrop". Anna and Susan collaborated together on fifteen fiction and children's books. Neither sister ever married, so they shared a house on Constitution Island right across from the famous West Point Military Academy.

The two sisters took a great interest in the Military Academy in which their uncle Thomas Warner was a chaplain and professor. As a result, they opened their home to the cadets and held Sunday School classes. Anna outlived her sickly sister by thirty years, and continued to run a very large Sunday School throughout her life. It was her invariable custom to write for her students a fresh hymn once a month. "Jesus Loves Me" was one of those monthly West Point hymns. Anna also gave the song to her sister Susan to use in the novel *Say and Seal*. In Susan's book, a Sunday School teacher sings 'Jesus Loves Me' to a sick pupil.

Great words without a great tune do not get very far in the musical world. Fortunately William Batchelder Bradbury stumbled across the "Jesus Loves Me" words, and wrote the now unforgettable tune. Thirteen years earlier, Bradbury had written the tune for the "Just as I am" hymn, which everyone associates with Billy Graham Crusades. In 1862, Bradbury found the "Jesus loves me" words in a best-selling 19th-century book, in which the words were spoken as a comforting poem to a dying child, John Fox. Along with his tune, Bradbury added his own chorus "Yes, Jesus loves me, Yes, Jesus Loves me…" Within months, this song raced across the hearts of children throughout North America, and eventually all the continents of the world.

Even after over 150 years, "Jesus Loves Me" is still the No. 1 spiritual song in the hearts of children around the world. Why is this? I believe that it is because all of us deep down need to know that God loves us. When I tell unchurched people that Jesus loves them, many of them genuinely thank me. One lady said: "Great…we can use lots of love". A man said: "Thanks…I'm going to need Him some day." Whatever situation we are in, we North American pirates need to know that the Lord really loves and cares for each of us.

TITUS 3:5-6 *"…he saved us, not because of righteous things we had done, but because of his mercy. He saved us through the washing of rebirth and renewal by the Holy Spirit, whom he poured out on us generously through Jesus Christ our Savior…"*

If God is not merciful, we are in deep trouble. Our sin and selfishness are so serious that our God and Saviour Jesus Christ had to die on the cross in our place. All of us need both rebirth and renewal to live a healthy life.

While leading a Renewal Mission at the Church of our Lord in Victoria, I went for an early morning walk to the ocean. There I saw an unforgettably beautiful pink-on-blue sky with a bright harvest moon, a gentle breeze, and chirping birds. Right in front of me was the Olympic Peninsula, Port Angeles with a partial lower cloud covering, seagulls and the rolling waves.

I was reminded on this walk of my Uncle Don Allen who had served as a career Naval Officer living in Victoria and in Halifax for most of his life. I loved my Uncle Don, and often visited him on holidays. Uncle Don retired to the Okanagan to tend a vineyard. In May 1982, I spent a week with my Uncle after my throat surgery was painfully postponed. Uncle Don's mom had just passed away, so he was spiritually searching. At the funeral, he had said to me: "If anyone deserved to go to heaven, it was Nana." I responded, saying "Nana was a great lady, but she is in heaven today not because of her goodness, but because of what Jesus did on the cross for her." While tending his vineyard, Uncle Don said to me that God was a good provider, but was off making other worlds. I said to Uncle Don: "You have God confused with your dad who was a good provider during the Great Depression, but worked seven days a week on night shift." Turning to the Vineyard, I explained John 15 to my uncle, that Jesus is the Vine and we are the branches. Jesus wants an intimate covenant relationship with us. Uncle Don was so excited that he spoke with me till 1am that night, ironically losing his voice. I had the sad privilege of taking my Uncle Don's funeral, and sharing how my Uncle came to know Jesus. Uncle Don is in heaven with his mom, not because of any righteous deeds that he has done, but because of what Jesus did on the cross for him.

Titus knew that healthy leadership is totally dependent on the renewal of the Holy Spirit. Without the power of the Holy Spirit, we are left to rowing our own boat when we could be sailing. Every pirate is looking for the wind to launch them on their next venture. It is so easy for us to resist the Spirit, quench the Spirit, grieve the Spirit, and vex the Spirit. God wants us to be filled and immersed with the Holy Spirit on a daily basis. The life-giving renewal of the Holy Spirit was foundational to the healthy transformation of Crete. Because Cretans were there at the Day of Pentecost, they never forgot that the outpouring of the Holy Spirit is indispensible for healthy Christian living. The Bible uses many images to describe the Holy Spirit, the third member of the Godhead: water, wind, fire and dove. All the images are fluid and life-giving. You cannot put the Holy Spirit in a box. John Calvin said that the smallest drop of the Spirit is, so to speak, like an everlasting fountain that never dries up.[243] We have been privileged at St. Simon's North Vancouver to offer the Alpha Course over thirty times. Nicky Gumbel, on the Holy Spirit Alpha weekend, says that there are no second-class Christians. Not all Christians speak in tongues, but all may. I am convinced that the gift of tongues is easily available today to all believers that are thirsty. We so often complicate things. Tongues, says Nicky Gumbel, is just a beginner's gift. Its purpose is to help strengthen our prayer lives. I have been using this gift since 1979 when Canon David Watson and my wife Janice prayed for the release of the Spirit in my life. Tongues, in my experience, seems to be helpful to releasing other spiritual gifts. It has been proven to be very useful in helping people get free from drug addiction. The Cretan ex-pirates would have been greatly helped by this healthy outpouring of the Holy Spirit.[244] God is waiting to do the same for North American pirates.

TITUS 3:7 *"so that, having been justified by his grace, we might become heirs having the hope of eternal life."*

Many North Americans have little if any idea what the term 'justified' might mean. 'Justified' means that we enter into a right relationship with God, just as if we had never sinned. 'Justified' means than we are forgiven by what Jesus did for us on the cross, taking our sins upon his own body. We are justified by grace through faith. The Anglican Article #11 clearly states that this is a 'most wholesome doctrine.' Justification by grace through faith is a healthy teaching that we all need to embrace. We cannot receive eternal life through our own works or deservings. It is a free gift that we either freely accept or freely reject. When we receive Christ by faith as our Lord and Saviour, he enters our life and we become heirs, having the hope of eternal life. For Cretan pirates, it was an amazing experience to realize that they could be forgiven and given a new beginning, no matter what evil things they had done in the past. No North American is either too good or too bad for justification by grace through faith. God is waiting for pirates to receive their inheritance through saying yes to his offer of life.

TITUS 3:8 *"This is a trustworthy saying. And I want you to stress these things, so that those who have trusted in God may be careful to devote themselves to doing what is good. These things are excellent and profitable for everyone."*

Let me stress an important truth: the excellent and profitable wisdom found in the book of Titus can be fully trusted. This is not well-meaning theory. You can take this to the bank. It will radically change your life if you actually put it into practice, if you take the prescribed spiritual medicine. The Cretan ex-pirates, infamous for being liars, evil brutes and lazy gluttons, became famous for their good works. All healthy followers of Christ need to be devoted to doing what is good. Goodness is neither powerless nor pretentious. Holistic goodness changes everything from the inside out. Alexander Fleming is a modern-day example of a healthy leader who devoted himself to doing good, which resulted in "excellent and profitable" goodness for everyone. When his picture turned up on the front cover of Time magazine, the byword stated "His penicillin will save more lives than war can spend". A vivid example of this "excellent and profitable goodness" was the usage of penicillin on D-Day to save 3,000 on Normandy Beach from deadly gangrene. Some researchers consider penicillin to be one of the key top-secret weapons that helped the Allies win World War II.

It is hard for our current generation fully to appreciate that before penicillin, even an infected pinprick or a tiny cut might be lethal. Hospitals were full of people with easily caught infections raging out of control. Children died regularly from scarlet fever, from infections of the bones, throat, stomach, or brain. It is no exaggeration to say that many of us reading this book would not be here today if it were not for the "excellent and profitable goodness" of antibiotics touching our extended families.

In 1881, Alexander Fleming was born in Ayrshire in the lowlands of southwestern Scotland. A playground accident smashed the bridge of his nose and left him looking like a battered boxer. Andre Maurois said that Fleming had those qualities which many attribute to the Scots: a capacity for hard and sustained work, a combative spirit which refuses to admit defeat, a steadfastness and loyalty which creates respect and affection, and a true humility which protects against pretentiousness and pride.

Affectionately called Little Flem, his gift of silence appeared to be inexhaustible. One colleague said that Fleming 'could be more eloquently silent than any man I have ever known.' His capacity for silence was only matched by his capacity for waiting – and for hanging on, an attribute that greatly helped him in his penicillin adventure.

The body's fight with infection was Fleming's abiding interest. One of Fleming's first breakthroughs was in the discovery of lysozyme, a natural antiseptic contained in human tears and saliva. Fleming's method of collecting lysozyme was to recruit a passing student or laboratory boy and drop lemon juice in his eye! Eventually Fleming switched to the use of egg white which has a stronger concentration of lysozyme.

Lysozyme, unfortunately, ended up being an embarrassment to Fleming because it proved useless in killing harmful diseases. As a result, his fellow colleagues mostly treated Fleming's later penicillin discovery as if it were another laboratory dead-end. Alexander Fleming always said, 'We shall hear more about lysozyme one day'. With thousands of scientific papers now written about it, the Russians use lysozyme for preserving caviar; doctors add lysozyme to cow-milk to reproduce the component structure of human milk, as well as for the treatment of eye and intestinal infections.

Fleming, being a 'packrat', never liked to throw anything away. One day, Fleming noticed a blue mould growing on one of his unwashed petri dishes. He seized the moment and changed the world forever. From that moment,

Fleming became obsessed with penicillin mould, even using his friends' moldy old shoes. Fleming showed amazing ingenuity in his makeshift creation of the first penicillin 'factory', employing devices like oilcans, biscuit tins, dustbins, bedpans, milk churns, and bookracks!

For twelve long years after his 1928 discovery of penicillin, Fleming faced skeptical indifference. Penicillin was a medical Cinderella that no one wanted to dance with. "The man of genius", wrote Lord Beaverbrook, "is often an egotist. When, as sometimes happens, he is simple and retiring, the world is inclined to underestimate his gifts..."

In 1937 Howard Florey and Ernst Chain of Oxford purified Fleming's lysozyme. From there, they purified Fleming's penicillin, making it stable, concentrated, and more useful. When Alexander Fleming turned up in Oxford, Chain was taken completely by surprise. He had thought that Fleming was dead! Fleming generously said of the two, "We all owe a lot to Florey, Chain and their co-workers. They did not initiate penicillin but they put it on the map as an effective drug."

By freeze-drying it at a low temperature with a neutral pH, Chain and Florey were able to purify penicillin to become a thousand times more powerful than Fleming's original mold. Once completely purified, penicillin became a million times stronger than at first!

By one biographer's account, Fleming was given 25 honorary degrees, 26 medals, 18 prizes, 13 decorations, the freedom of 15 cities and boroughs, and honorary membership in 89 academies and societies. Both Florey and Fleming were knighted in 1944, and in 1945 Fleming, Florey and Chain were jointly given the Nobel Prize for Physiology and Medicine. Medical centers, research institutes, and even a moon crater were named in honour of the beloved 'father' of penicillin. It meant a lot to Fleming as a Scot when he was elected as Rector of Edinburgh University in 1951. When Fleming received an ovation at a Spanish bullfight, 20,000 fans broke out into mass hysteria. The famous Spanish scientist Don Gregorio Maranon said of Fleming that "God selected him to carry out the greatest miracle which humanity has ever seen".

Yet despite all the honours showered on Fleming, fame did not spoil him. He remained a simple humble man, not even bothering to patent penicillin for personal profit. When Fleming was asked to what he attributed his success, he said: "I can only suppose that God wanted penicillin, and that this was his reason for creating Alexander Fleming." Like Fleming, we need to devote ourselves to doing good through restoring health in the lives of others.

TITUS 3:9 *"But avoid foolish controversies and genealogies and arguments and quarrels about the law, because these are unprofitable and useless."*

Pirates love to argue and joust with each other for the fun of it. For many North Americans, religion is a blood sport. They love to argue about non-essentials, because for them everything is essential. They are painfully right and everyone else is hopelessly deceived. While we do need to stand up for the essentials of the Gospel, we also are wise to not be drawn into useless, endless arguments. Ex-pirates may be tempted to fight and argue rather than to pray and act. Many anxious, angry North Americans love to argue about the second coming, the sacraments, and especially sacred songs. Worship wars have ripped apart countless North American churches. Paul clearly tells Titus that this is a distraction from strengthening a new genera-tion of healthy leaders. Do not go there. This is a dead end. Such quarrelling is unprofitable and useless. It will keep you from finishing well, from mak-ing your major life contribution. John Calvin said that "such people never run out of words as they always have new strength from their wickedness, so they never tire of fighting."[245] That is why Paul said that they are warped, sinful and self-condemned. Our North American addiction to schism often becomes my dogmatism chasing your catechism. We need to be careful that we do not define ourselves by what we oppose. Stay focused on Christ. Jesus cautioned us in Matthew 7:6 not to cast our pearls foolishly before others. Choose your battles wisely. Stand firm for biblical truth and sound doctrine without being obnoxiously aggressive.

TITUS 3:14 *"Our people must learn to devote themselves to doing what is good in order that they may provide for daily necessities and not live unproductive lives."*

Even in the midst of sending personal greetings and asking for hospitality for fellow workers, Paul returns to the heart of his message. The Cret-an ex-pirates need to turn from selfishness to goodness. They were to do their best and do everything they can to make a lasting difference. Instead of being plundering pirates, they are to be producing and providing for themselves and their families. Only by the washing of regeneration and the renewal of the Holy Spirit could an entire society shift to become a King-dom-based culture. If this could happen to Cretan pirates, this can happen in North America.

Because our hearts are deceitful, it is very difficult to see and acknow-ledge one's own pirate tendencies. We North Americans would rather point the finger at other people's piracies. Only those pirates who admit the toxic truth about themselves can move towards good health. Who were the real pirates in the American Revolution: the British, the Americans, or even both?

Whether one was a pirate or a legal privateer was often in the eye of the beholder. The British had a long history of employing government-licensed privateers like Sir Francis Drake who rescued England from the 1588 Span-ish Armada. Sir Francis Drake is remembered by the Spanish as the pirate dragon, El Drako. Such pirate tendencies re-emerged during the American Revolution. Benjamin Franklin protested to the British Lord Admiral Howe about the pirate behaviour of his British military:

> ...the most wanton barbarity and cruelty burnt our defenseless towns in the midst of winter, excited the savages to massacre our peaceful farmers, and our slaves to murder their masters, and is even now bringing foreign mercenaries to deluge our settlements with blood.[246]

In 1778, while ambassador to France, Benjamin Franklin raised up a pri-vateer fleet to capture British sailors and use them to exchange for the Americans held by the British in very difficult conditions.[247] Around 800 American privateer ships were commissioned, resulting in the loss of around 600 British ships. Between ten to thirty thousand American privateers were imprisoned by the British and treated as common pirates treasonously re-belling against King George III. At the end of the American Revolution, Franklin unsuccessfully attempted to include in the Peace Treaty a ban on future privateering.[248]

Like Titus, Benjamin Franklin taught the American people to devote themselves to doing what is good, to live productive lives. I remember as a young child being taught Benjamin Franklin's proverb: 'Early to bed, early to rise, makes a person healthy, wealthy and wise. As a brilliant philosopher, he shared wisdom through short pithy sayings like 'He that lies down with dogs shall rise up with fleas.' Many of Franklin's sayings are so well known that people confuse them as coming from the Bible. 'God helps those who help themselves' is from Franklin, not from Jesus.[249]

Many of his sayings were published in Poor Richard's Almanack, a book series that has had a profound impact on North American culture and identity. Some would say that the middle class dreams and ideals can be traced back directly to Benjamin Franklin's homespun philosophy. Many of us unknowingly quote Benjamin Franklin on a regular basis: haste makes waste; no pain, no gain; and nothing is certain but death and taxes. Most of Franklin's sayings were about encouraging diligence, honesty, industry and temperance. Franklin saw the Judeo-Christian ethic as "the best the world ever saw or is likely to see."[250] Not everyone liked Benjamin Franklin. DH Lawrence said: "I do not like him....that barbed wire moral enclosure that Poor Richard rigged up....Benjamin Franklin tried to take away my wholeness and my dark forest, my freedom."[251]

Benjamin Franklin's father had intended that his son Benjamin train to be a clergyman, but lacked the resources to do so. Instead Benjamin became a printer and an inventor. Benjamin Franklin is world-famous for his kite experiments with lightning, proving that lightning was made up of electricity. Some see him as the world's first electrician. While visiting England, he attached his latest invention, the lightning rod, to St Paul's Cathedral.[252] He also created hot-water pipes to warm up the chilly British House of Commons. Other significant Franklin inventions were bifocals and the Franklin stove.[253]

Benjamin Franklin was far ahead of his time in terms of understanding workplace toxicity. As a printer, he discovered that newspaper workers were being poisoned through handling hot lead type, causing stiffness and paralysis. Franklin found out that this lead poisoning was also affecting glazers, type-founders, plumbers, potters, white-lead makers and painters.[254]

Benjamin Franklin was so successful in business that he retired at age 42 and devoted the rest of his life to public service. He moved to England twice in order to help the relationship between England and its American colonies. While in England, Franklin wrote most of his autobiography at the home of the Bishop of St. Asaph, Jonathan Shipley. His book became the world's most popular autobiography, and has been translated into most major languages. Franklin's autobiography was the one book which Davy Crockett had when slaughtered at the Alamo.[255]

Despite his being a strong Royalist, Benjamin Franklin ended up being resented by the British House of Lords who publicly humiliated him for his efforts to bring reconciliation between England and its American colonies. This was Franklin's tipping point where he became a strong advocate for Independence. As America's first postmaster general, Franklin was also put in charge of establishing the first US currency. In the aftermath of the Boston Tea Party, Franklin recommended that Americans give up tea drinking as a way to fund their new government.[256] The constitution's phrase 'We hold these truths to be self-evident' was the direct result of Franklin's editing.[257]

Franklin was the only one to sign all four of the USA's founding papers: the Declaration of Independence, the treaty with France, the peace accord with Britain, and the Constitution. His unsuccessful proposal for the American Great Seal was to have Pharaoh being swallowed by the Red Sea, along with the words 'Rebellion to Tyrants is Obedience to God.'[258]

Franklin's greatest popularity was among the French who lined the streets when he entered Paris as the USA's first foreign diplomat. The French saw him as a simple frontier sage, and promptly put his likeness everywhere, causing the French King to become very jealous.[259] Without Franklin's winning the moral and financial support of the French, it is doubtful that the United States would have survived.

Franklin was a very complicated, even tragic individual with strong approach/avoidance tendencies. He loved the United States but spent most of his last years in England and then France. His relations with the opposite sex were muddled and confused. He loved his wife and family but was away more than at home and suffered a painful split with his son William over politics.

Despite Franklin's reputation as a religious skeptic, he went out of his way in his newspaper to promote the Rev George Whitfield who led North America's first Great Awakening in 1739-1741. As a scientist, he was amazed that Whitfield's voice could be heard without amplification by over 30,000 people at one time. Franklin published all of Whitfield's books and posted his sermons on the front page of his Philadelphia Gazette. This renewal of the Holy Spirit clearly impacted Franklin. Whitfield wrote to Franklin, saying: "As you have made a pretty considerable progress in the mysteries of electricity, I would now humbly recommend to your diligent unprejudiced pursuit and study the mystery of the new-birth. It is a most important, interesting study, and when mastered, will richly answer and repay you for all your pains."[260] His friend Whitfield knew that the washing of regeneration could change any North American's heart.

After jealous clergy closed their pulpits to Whitfield, Franklin and other trustees built a large hall where Whitfield could preach. Franklin commented: "It was wonderful to see the change soon made in the manners of our inhabitants." After the revival ended, Franklin converted the hall into the Academy of Philadelphia which later became the University of Pennsylvania.

As Governor of Pennsylvania, Franklin in 1748 proposed a day of fasting and prayer. In 1778, Franklin wrote to the French Government, saying: "Whoever shall introduce into public affairs the principals of primitive Christianity will change the face of the world.", recommending that every

French home have a Bible and newspaper, and a good school in every district.[261]

At the 1787 American Constitutional Convention, Franklin commented: "the longer I live, the more convincing proofs I see of this truth—that God governs in the affairs of men. And if a sparrow cannot fall to the ground without His notice, is it probable that an empire can rise without His aid?" On that basis, Franklin arranged that prayers led by local clergy would be held each morning before Assembly business. Franklin said: "If I had ever before been an atheist, I should now have been convinced of the Being and government of a Deity!"[262]

Franklin was passionate about finishing well and making amends. To that end, he died viewing a picture of the Day of Judgement by his bedside. Three years before his death, Franklin became the President of the *Pennsylvania Society for Promoting the Abolition of Slavery*. As a young man, he was a slaveowner and sold slavery ads in his *Pennyslvania Gazette* newspaper. Shortly before his death in 1790, Franklin's last public act was to unsuccessfully petition the US Congress to abolish slavery. In particular, the petition implored that the US Congress "devise means for removing the Inconsistency from the Character of the American People…promote mercy and justice toward this distressed Race…for discouraging every species of Traffick in the Persons of our fellow men." Franklin stated in the petition that:

> mankind are all formed by the same Almighty being, alike objects of his Care, and equally designed for the Enjoyment of Happiness the Christian religion teaches us to believe, and the Political Creed of America fully coincides with the Position.

Ten percent of Philadelphians and over seventeen percent of all the four million Americans were trapped in slavery.[263] After a fiery debate, Franklin's anti-slavery petition was referred to a select committee and then tragically tabled. Imagine how the USA's history might have been different if this act of piracy had been abolished in 1790, rather than seventy-three years later by Abraham Lincoln during a bloody civil war. Imagine what might happen if a modern day Benjamin Franklin would speak out for the rights of our youngest and oldest North Americans in this age of dehumanizing abortion and euthanasia. I have to believe that justice and human rights will eventually come for our unborn and elderly North American neighbours. There must be a more humane solution than the current North American status quo.

Franklin memorably commented: "Think of three things: Whence you came, where you are going, and to whom you must give account."[264] May each of us, like Benjamin Franklin, be willing to be accountable to God in choosing the way of health, the way of life, the way of godliness.

My prayer for those reading this book is that you will be not just hearers of the word, but doers of the word. We need to put the forgotten book of Titus into practice. Holistically healthy leaders are key to transforming the world around us, to putting into order what is left unfinished. It is time to say no to the toxic piracy that has become normalized in North America. Our piracy, just like that of the 1st century Cretans, needs to be brought to the foot of the cross. Jesus can actually transform us by the washing of regeneration and the renewing of the Holy Spirit. Putting the book of Titus into practice will revolutionize the holistic health of yourselves, your church, your community, your nation. We North Americans need to become convergently healthy and godly in body, mind and spirit. Applying these holistic principles from the ancient island of Crete will strengthen a new generation of healthy North American leaders. Imagine what our world would look like if it became filled with unstoppable world-changing Tituses. Imagine if we North Americans actually repented of our pirate ways, of our idolatry and immorality. I challenge you as North Americans to choose the healthy way of Christlikeness. Say no to piracy and yes to Christ. Choose to live out a 21st century Jesus revolution. Revival and new life is coming to North America and to the ends of the earth. Choose life as healthy leaders that you and your children may live. Join me in this revolution from death to life.

The Rev. Dr. Ed Hird
Rector, St. Simon's Church North Vancouver
edhird.com

Select Bibliography

Barclay, William, *The Daily Study Bible: The Letters to Timothy, Titus and Philemon*, (GR Welch Co. Ltd., Burlington, Ontario. 1956, 1975)

Barrett, CK, *The Pastoral Epistles*, (Oxford University Press, 1963)

Baxter, Richard, *The Reformed Pastor*, (Monergism Books)

Baxter, Richard, *The Saint's Everlasting Rest*, 1650, (Regent College Publishing, 2004)

Bartling, Victor and Moellering, H. Armin, *1 Timothy, 2 Timothy, Titus*, (Concordia Publishing House, Saint Louis, Missouri, 1970).

Bassler, Jouette, *1 Timothy, 2 Timothy, Titus*, (Abingdon New Testament Commentaries, 1996).

Blaiklock, EM, *The Pastoral Epistles: a Study Guide*, (Zondervan Publishing House, Grand Rapids, Michigan, 1972).

Botting, Douglas, *The Seafarers: The Pirates*, (Time-Life Books Inc., 1978).

Bratcher, Robert, *A Translator's Guide to Paul's Letters to Timothy and to Titus*, (United Bible Societies, London, England, 1983).

Briscoe, Stuart, *Purifying the Church: What God Expects of You and Your Church: A Topical Commentary on Titus*, (Regal Books, GL Publications, 1987).

Calvin, John, *1 & 2 Timothy & Titus*, (The Crossway Classic Commentaries, Wheaton, Illinois, 1998

Finch, Michael, *GK Chesterton: Biography*, (Harper Collins, USA, 1986).

Collins, Raymond F, *1 & 2 Timothy and Titus*, (Westminster John Knox Press, Louisville, Kentucky, 2002).

Cordingly, David, *Under the Black Flag: The Romance and the Reality of Life among the Pirates*, (Random House, New York, 1995)

Cottrell, Leonard, *The Bull of Minos*, (Pan Books Ltd, London, England, 1951, 1961).

Dibelius, Martin and Conzelmann, Hans, translated by Philip Buttolph and Yarbro, Adlea, *A Commentary on the Pastoral Epistles*, (Fortress Press, Philadelphia, 1972, 1984).

Easton, Burton Scott, *The Pastoral Epistles*, (SCM Press, London, England, 1948).

Enslin, Morton, *Letters to the Churches: 1st and 2nd Timothy, Titus*, (Lutterworth Press, London, 1963).

Fee, Gordon, *1 & 2 Timothy, Titus, New International Biblical Commentary*, (Hendrickson Publishers, Peabody, Massachusetts, 1984, 1988).

Fodor's: Exploring the Greek Islands, (Fodor's Travel Publications Inc, 2004).

France, Dick, *Timothy, Titus and Hebrews: The People's Bible Commentary*, (BRF, Oxford, UK, 2001).

Getz, Gene A, *Saying No When You'd Rather Say Yes: Making Choices Based on Titus*, (Regal Books, Ventura, California, 1978).

Griffiths, Michael, *Timothy and Titus*, (Baker Books, Grand Rapids, Michigan, 1996).

Guthrie, Donald, *The Pastoral Epistles*, (Eerdmans Publishing Co., Grand Rapids, Michigan, 1957, 1974).

Guthrie, Donald, *The Pastoral Epistles and the Mind of Paul*, (The Tyndale Press, London, England, 1955).

Hanson, AT, *The New Century Bible Commentary: The Pastoral Epistles*, , (Eerdmans Publishing Company, Grand Rapids, Michigan, 1982).

Harding, Mark, *What are they saying about the Pastoral Epistles?*, (Paulist Press, Mahwah, New Jersey, 2001).

Harris, Graham, *Treasure and Intrigue: the Legacy of Captain Kidd, Dundurn Press*, (Toronto, Ontario, 2002).

Hendriksen, William, *Commentary on 1ˢᵗ & 2ⁿᵈ Timothy and Titus*, (The Banner of Truth Trust, 1959).

Houden, JL, *The Pastoral Epistles*, (The Pelican New Testament Commentaries, 1976).

Horwood, Harold and Butts, Ed, *Pirates & Outlaws of Canada: 1610-1932*, (Doubleday Canada Limited, Toronto, Ontario, 1984).

Hultgren, Arland J., *I-II Timothy, Titus*, (Augsburg Publishing House, Minneapolis, Minnesota, 1984).

Hutchinson, RW, *Prehistoric Crete*, (Penguin Books, London, England, 1962, 1963).

The Interpreter's Dictionary of the Bible, (Abingdon Press, Nashville, Tennessee, 1962).

Insight Guides: Greek Islands, (Discovery Channel, APA Publications, 2003).

Ironside, HA, *Timothy, Titus and Philemon*, (Loizeaux Brothers, Neptune, New Jersey, 1947, 1972).

Johnson, Luke Timothy, *Letters to Paul's Delegates: 1 Timothy, 2 Timothy, Titus*, (Trinity Press International, Valley Forge, Pennsylvania, 1996).

Johnson, Philip C, *The Epistles to Titus and Philemon*, (Baker Book House, Grand Rapids, Michigan, 1966).

Jones, E. Stanley, *Victorious Living*, (Abingdon Press, New York, NY, 1936).

Karris, Robert J., *The Pastoral Epistles*, (OFM, Michael Glazier, Inc, Wilmington, Delaware, 1979).

Kelly, JND, *A Commentary on the Pastoral Epistles*, (Harper and Row, New York, NY, 1963).

Kelly, William, *An Exposition of the Epistle of Paul to Titus and of that to Philemon*, (Believers Bookshelf, Sunbury, Pennsylvania, 1968).

Kelsey, Harry, *Sir Francis Drake: the Queen's Pirate*, (Yale University Press, New Haven, USA, 1998).

Keyes, Dick, *Seeing Through Cynicism*, (IVP, Westmont, Illinois, 2006).

Knight III, George W, *The Pastoral Epistles: A Commentary on the Greek Text, Eerdmans Publishing Company*, (Grand Rapids, Michigan, & Paternoster Press, Carlisle, England, 1992).

Konstam, Angus, *The History of Pirates*, (The Lyons Press, New York, NY, 1999).

Lea, Thomas and Griffin Jr, Hayne P., *The New American Commentary, 1 & 2 Timothy & Titus*, (Broadman Press, Nashville, Tennessee, 1992).

Lewis, CS, *Prince Caspian*, (Puffin Book, London, UK, 1951).

The Life of the Reverend Richard Baxter, (London, 1696).

Lincoln, Margarette, *The Pirate's Handbook*, (Cobblehill Books, New York, NY, 1995).

Maclaren, Alexander, *II Timothy, Titus, Philemon and Hebrews*, (Hodder and Stoughton, London, UK, MCMX).

Martin, Hugh, *Puritanism and Richard Baxter*, (SCM Press, London, 1954).

Milne, Douglas, *Focus on the Bible 1, 2 Timothy & Titus* , (Christian Focus Publications, Great Britain, 1996).

Morris, Leon, *Scripture Union Bible Study Books: 1 Timothy-James,* (Eerdmans Publishing Company, Grand Rapids, Michigan, 1969).

Oden, Thomas C., *First and Second Timothy and Titus: Interpretation*, (John Knox Press, Louisville, Kentucky, 1989).

Packer, JI, *Oxford Doctoral Thesis*: "Redemption and Restoration of Man in the Thought of Richard Baxter", (Regent College Publishing, 2003).

Platon, Nicholas, *Crete,* (Frederick Muller Limited, London, Nagel Publishers, 1966).

Platon, Nicholas, *Zakros: the Discovery of a Lost Palace of Ancient Crete,* (Charles Scribner's Sons, New York, 1971).

Plummer, Alfred, *the Pastoral Epistles,* (Funk and Wagnalls Company, New York, USA, 1900).

Powicke, Frederick, *A Life of Richard Baxter,* MCMXXIV.

Quinn, Jerome D., *The Letter to Titus,* (The Anchor Bible, Doubleday, New York, NY, 1990).

Sanders, Richard, *If a Pirate I Must Be…: the true story of Bartholomew Roberts: King of the Caribbean,* (Aurum Press Ltd, 2007).

Sherry, Frank, *Raiders and Rebels: the Golden Age of Piracy,* (Hearst Marine Books, New York, NY, 1986).

Shoemaker, Sam, *If I be Lifted Up,* 1931.

Simpson, E.K., *The Pastoral Epistles,* (The Tyndale Press, London, UK, 1954).

Soo-Inn Tan, *Leadership Qualifications in the Pastoral Epistles: Criteria and Context,* Masters of Theology Thesis, (Regent College, 1985)

Stam, Cornelius R., *Commentary on the Pastoral Epistles of Paul the Apostle, Berean Bible Society,* (Chicago, Illinois, 1983).

Stott, John, *Guard the Truth: the message of 1 Timothy & Titus,* (Intervarsity Press, 1996).

Talty, Stephan, *Empire of Blue Water,* (Crown Publishing Group, Random House Inc, New York, NY, 2007).

Towner, Philip H., *1-2 Timothy & Titus,* (Intervarsity Press, Downers Grove, Illinois, 1994).

Towner, Philip H., *The Letters to Timothy and Titus: The New International Commentary on the New Testament,* (Wm Eerdmans Publishing Co., Grand Rapids, Michigan, 2006).

Unger, Merrill F, *Unger's Bible Dictionary,* (Moody Press, Chicago, 1957, 1973).

Unsworth, Barry, *Crete,* (National Geographic Society, Washington, DC, 2004).

Ward, Ronald A., *Commentary of 1st & 2nd Timothy & Titus,* (Word Books, Waco, Texas, 1974).

Woodard, Colin, *The Republic of Pirates,* (Harcourt Inc, Orlando, Florida, 2007).

Wright, Tom, *Paul for Everyone: The Pastoral Epistles,* (SPCK, London, England, 2003).

Wunderlich, Hans George, *The Secret of Crete,* (Macmillan Publishing Co, Inc., New York, NY, 1974).

Endnotes

1   The 'Strengthening a New Generation of Healthy Leaders' book series will include 1) the Titus book: *Restoring Health: Body, Mind and Spirit.* 2) Strengthening Marriage book: *Strengthening the Marriages of a New Generation of Healthy Leaders* 3) Incarnational Renewal book: *Strengthening the New Generation of Leaders in Healthy Incarnational Renewal* 4) Power of Jesus to Heal Today book: *Strengthening the New Generation of Leaders in Healing* 5) Emotional Cutoff book: *Strengthening the New Generation of Healthy Leaders Through Family Systems Wisdom* 6) Devotional Commentary on 1 Corinthians: *Strengthening the New Generation of Healthy Leaders Through Small Groups.*

2   Terry B Walling, *Stuck!,* (ChurchSmart Resources, 2008), p. XIII "Without transitions, and the paradigm shifts that occur, Christ followers would stay stuck!"

3   This Pre-Lambeth Leadership Conference was jointly sponsored by Anglican Renewal Ministries/ARM and SOMA/Sharing of Ministries Abroad. I was serving as the Chair of ARM Canada.

4   Freda Meadows ministers with the International New Wine Director Rev Bruce Collins http://www.new-wine.org; Ten years later, the Rev Freda gave further insight into the 1998 Canterbury prophecy, saying:
     "...the underlying thrust was to trust God for the outcome of the plans He had in using you. While you were to do all that was necessary, it was not for you to try and make anything happen. But you were to follow the Lord's leading using the gifts and skills He gave in the best way you knew and through what you had learned as your experience grew."

5   http://poetry.poetryx.com/poems/784/

6   "African Christians? They're just a step up from witchcraft," What Bishop Spong had to say about his fellow Christians, John Spong interviewed by Andrew Carey, *Church of England Newspaper,* July 10th 1998. Newspaper & Andrew Carey. "They've moved out of animism into a very superstitious kind of Christianity. They've yet to face the intellectual revolution of Copernicus and Einstein that we've had to face in the developing world. That's just not on their radar screen."

7   Doug LeBlanc, Lambeth, 1998, "Episcopal Dissidents, African Allies", Dr Miranda Hassett, University of North Carolina, Chapel Hill, http://anglicanhistory.org/academic/hassett2004.pdf

8   On October 17th Wednesday 2008 while at the Anglican Coalition Clergy Retreat at Cedar Springs, I received a distinct impression from the Lord while in deep quiet group prayer: "Yes, it is Titus." While attending the Henry Wright 'Be in Health' conference, I heard a still small voice saying: "Write 3rd book on Titus for North American Audience."

9   1 Corinthians 14:3

10   1 Thessalonians 5: 19-21: Do not put out the Spirit's fire; do not treat prophecies with contempt. Test everything. Hold on to the good. Avoid every kind of evil.; 1 Corinthians 13:9.

11   1 Timothy 1:18, 4:14

12   Titus is listed by name in 2 Cor 2:13; 7:6, 13, 14; 8:6, 16, 23; 12:18; Gal 2:1, 3; 2 Tim 4:10; Titus 1:4

13   Galatians 2:3; George W Knight III, The Pastoral Epistles: A Commentary on the Greek Text, Eerdmans Publishing Company, Grand Rapids, Michigan, & Paternoster Press, Carlisle, England, 1992, p. 8

14   Angus Konstam, *The History of Pirates,* (The Lyons Press, New York, NY, 1999), p. 24 "In the 10th Century BC, the Minoan civilization was overrun by Dorian Greeks, who engaged in piratical raids using Cretan cities as bases. In Homer's Odyssey, the Cretans were described as pirates. Crete continued to be a pirate base for almost 800 years..."

15   *Battle for the Soul of Canada* book, 2006, 2007, http://www.battleforthesoulofcanada.blogspot.org

16   George W. Knight III, GK p. 21 "...In 1812 Eichhorn extended Schleirmacher's judgement to all three Pastoral Epistles on the basis of divergent religious language (Eichhorn, Einleitung, III/1, 137ff.)...The position became widespread in the English-speaking world with the publication in 1921 of Harrison's well known book 'The Problem of the Pastorals", which advanced its case on the basis of detailed linguistic and stylistic analyses."

17   C.K. Barrett, *The Pastoral Epistles,* (Oxford University Press, 1963), p. 3,4, 9; Eusebius, *Historia Ecclesiastic* III. iii. 5.

18   George W Knight III, p. 3: "The earliest known use of the term was by Berdot, writing in 1703 and referring to Titus. It was applied to all three letters in a work by Anton published posthumously in 1753-55. "

19   Titus 3:8, NIV.

20   1 Corinthians 16:10, NIV "If Timothy comes, see that he has nothing to fear while he is with you…" In some ways, Canada's personality is Timothy, and our USA sister country is a Titus.

21   Walter Isaacson, *Steve Jobs* (Simon & Schuster, New York, NY, 2011), p. 145.

22   Andy Hertzfeld, "A Rich Neighbor Named Xerox", November 1983; Martin Burke, *Pirates of the Silicon Valley* movie, 1999. http://www.folklore.org/StoryView.py?story=A_Rich_Neighbor_Named_Xerox.txt (Accessed Feb 1st 2014)

23   William Barclay, *The Daily Study Bible: The Letters to Timothy, Titus and Philemon*, (GR Welch Co. Ltd., Burlington, Ontario. 1956, 1975), p. 232

24   Gene A Getz, *Saying No When You'd Rather Say Yes: Making Choices Based on Titus*, Regal Books, Ventura, California, 1978, p. 29

25   Michael Griffiths, *Timothy and Titus*, Baker Books, Grand Rapids, Michigan, 1996, p. 128

26   *Alcoholics Anonymous Book*, Fourth Edition, 2001, Alcoholic Anonymous World Services Inc, New York City, p. 58

27   Gene Getz, p. 30 "Titus stood firm for what was right…Titus was loyal – not for loyalty's sake but because it was the right thing to do. He stood for the truth, no matter what it cost him personally."

28   George W Knight III, p. 287; Iliad 2:649

29   2 Corinthians 8:17

30   Michael Griffiths, p. 161 "Four times in 2 Corinthians 8:16-24 the same Greek root word occurs in describing Titus, translated variously as 'concern' (v. 16), 'enthusiasm' (vs 17) and 'zealous' and 'confidence' (vs. 22).

31   One's soul or psyche is one's mind.

32   Philip H. Towner, *The Letters to Timothy and Titus*, (The New International Commentary on the New Testament, Wm Eerdmans Publishing Co., Grand Rapids, Michigan, 2006), p. 664

33   Bishop Silas Ng, *Discipler123 Blog*, August 6th 2011 "The last time I saw Uncle John in July 2009 he told me, "Silas, if you want me to conclude the most important thing I've got in my whole life, it is just one word, and that is—Christlikeness!" http://discipler123.blogspot.ca/2011/08/day-155-see-you-in-heaven-uncle-john.html

34   Tom Wright, *Paul for Everyone: The Pastoral Epistles*, SPCK, London, England, 2003. p. 141

35   Isaiah 40:31

36   Stephanie Smith, "Boomeritis': A generation of sports injuries", CNN, Thursday, May 15, 2003 http://www.cnn.com/2003/HEALTH/05/15/boomeritis/index.html?_s=PM:HEALTH (accessed Dec 12th 2013)

37   Benjamin Franklin, *Poor Richard's Almanac*, 1746

38   Psalm 103:4

39   Dec 31st 2011 Twitter, Mark Batterson, Lead Pastor, National Community Church (theaterchurch.com) in Washington DC.

40   http://www.quotegarden.com/exercise.html (accessed August 23rd 2014)

41   http://www.goodreads.com/quotes/show/175702 (accessed July 4th 2011)

42   Dr E Stanley Jones, *The Way to Power and Poise*, Abingdon Press, 1949, p. 152

43   Dr. Brene Brown, *The Power of Vulnerability*, TED Talk, June 2010, https://www.ted.com/talks/brene_brown_on_vulnerability/transcript (accessed June 22nd 2014).

44   Colin James Cross, MCS Regent College Thesis ""Agnes Sanford and the Heritage of Inner Healing", 1986, p. 41

45 Oct 20th 2009 Tuesday evening,Lee Grady, (then) Editor of *Charisma Magazine* came to West Point Christian Assembly, giving me a prophecy: "Lord, we thank you now in the name of Jesus for the ministry of healing. Lord, there is already a flow of healing but there is something new and fresh. And Lord, there is a well that you want to release in this brother and this congregation. I see a well opening up. I see a well of healing. And it's a well that people, Lord, are going to talk about. People are going to begin to say: 'Have you heard about that? Have you been there? Have you experienced that?' Because there is something that is about to break out, something that is about to flow, a fresh spring of healing water flowing. It's healing to the body and it's healing to the emotions. It's healing to the mind and there's just a total healing anointing: body, soul, spirit, that's flowing out of these people, and flowing into needy hurting places. And it's going to be something that people will talk about and bring people to, and the word's going to get out: 'Did you know that there is healing in that place?' And the enemy tried to dam this up, and he tried to throw garbage into it and stop it. But, Lord, we decree tonight in Jesus' name that this spring will spring up afresh, in the name of Jesus, and that nothing, Lord, will stop it from flowing. The enemy tried to bring a pollution in there, but we just say in the name of Jesus that, Lord, just as those wells were cleaned out in the days of Jacob, Lord, that this will happen in this place and that what the enemy strategized in the past will be unraveled. Lord, we say that this man of God will raise up teams of healers in the name of Jesus. We say that teams will flow together and let them go forth to the four corners. Lord, let them be raised up and trained as teams, Lord, to bring body, soul and spirit restoration. Thank you, Lord Jesus, for that call of God on this man's life. In Jesus name. Thank you Lord. Thank you Lord. Thank you Lord."

46 Eusebius, *Church History* 3.4.6, p. 136.

47 Alpha & Omega, http://www.alpha-omegaonline.com/road/heraklion.htm "In 1363... (The Cretans) lowered the flag of the Republic of St. Mark (Venice) and raised on the bell tower of the church the flag of the Republic of St. Titus." (accessed Dec 16th 2013).

48 Orthodox Church of Crete http://www.iak.gr/gr/index.html

49 Angus Konstam, *The History of Pirates*, (The Lyons Press, New York, NY, 1999), p. 8.

50 "Piracy in International Law is the crime of robbery or other act of violence for private ends on the high seas or in the air above the seas, committed by the captain or crew of a ship or aircraft outside the normal jurisdiction of any nation, and without authority from any government" http://www. thepirateking.com/terminology/definition_pirate.htm (accessed Dec 14th 2013).; The international definition of piracy is part of the 1982 "United Nations Convention on the Law of the Sea" or UNCLOS. The following text is taken directly from Article 101 of the UNCLOS. "Piracy consists of any of the following acts: (a) any illegal acts of violence or detention, or any act of depredation, committed for private ends by the crew or the passengers of a private ship or a private aircraft, and directed:(i) on the high seas, against another ship or aircraft, or against persons or property on board such ship or aircraft;(ii) against a ship, aircraft, persons or property in a place outside the jurisdiction of any State; (b) any act of voluntary participation in the operation of a ship or of an aircraft with knowledge of facts making it a pirate ship or aircraft;(c) any act inciting or of intentionally facilitating an act described in sub-paragraph (a) or (b). http://maritime.about.com/od/Safety/a/Definition-of-Piracy.htm (accessed Dec 14th 2013)

51 'Downtown Atlanta could get pirate museum', by Leon Stafford, The Atlanta Journal-Constitution, Oct 16th 2009, http://www.ajc.com/news/atlanta/downtown-atlanta-could-get-164610.html

52 Douglas Botting, The Seafarers: The Pirates, Time-Life Books Inc., 1978, p. 22

53 Mark Twain, *Life on the Mississippi*, http://www.gutenberg.org/files/245/245-h/245-h.htm, 1883.

54 Mark Twain's Autobiography, a chapter published in the North American Review, Sept. 1907.

55 Vancouver Sun, September 27th 2008, *Somali pirates demand $35 million ransom for military ship* http://www.canada.com/vancouversun/news/story.html?id=21d03049-e33b-4d78-91e6-f5c35e8446c3

56 Dr E. Stanley Jones, *Abundant Living*, Abingdon, Nashville, 1942, p. 362

57 1 Corinthians 1

58 Douglas Milne, *Focus on the Bible 1, 2 Timothy & Titus* , 1996, Christian Focus Publications, Great Britain, p. 199

59 Barry Unsworth, *Crete*, (National Geographic Society, Washington, DC, 2004), p. 160, "Cretan music: the beauty of the island and the indomitable spirit of the people...the refusal to submit"

60 Dr Philip Towner, Commentary on Timothy and Titus, p. 40

61 8,336 km²

62 Michael Griffiths, *Timothy and Titus*, (Baker Books, Grand Rapids, Michigan), 1996, p. 126; (2425 m)

63 Barry Unsworth, *Crete*, p. 12

64 Insight Guides: p. 281, p. 286 "…Claimed by many Greeks to be the most authentic of the islands…"

65 Unsworth, p. 12

66 Didorus 5:77:3

67 Griffiths, p. 126

68 The Interpreter's Dictionary of the Bible, p. 791 "ccording to biblical tradition, the Philistines came originally from Caphtor, the Hebrew name for Crete (Jeremiah 47"4; Amos 9:7)…it was buttressed by the fact that part of the Philistine coast was called 'the Cretan Negeb' 'Negeb of the Cherethites' (1 Samuel 30:14)"

69 Griffiths, p. 126

70 During the 200 years of Turkish occupation from about 1700 to 1900, the Cretans waged 350 revolutions. In 1821, the Greek War of Independence began, with extensive Cretan involvement. Several Cretan bishops were executed as ringleaders. It was not until 1898 when Crete became free, remaining so until 1913, when it chose to join Greece.

71 Hans George Wunderlich, *The Secret of Crete*, (Macmillan Publishing Co, Inc., New York, NY, 1974), p. 4

72 CS Lewis, *The Lion, the Witch and the Wardrobe*, HarperCollins, 1950

73 Plato, (425-347 BC); Hans George Wunderlich, p. 281 "Karl Kerenyi speaks of the 'honeyed' Zeus of the dead who receives the veneration of the living in the form of a serpent. Nectar and ambrosia make up the traditional food of the gods on Olympus."

74 Hans George Wunderlich, p. 283

75 Hans George Wunderlich, p. 283

76 http://en.wikipedia.org/wiki/Greek_War_of_Independence "Egyptians administered the island (of Crete), such as the Egyptian-Albanian Giritli Mustafa Naili Pasha." (accessed Feb 2009)

77 Acts 2:11

78 Titus 1:5 NIV; KJV "set in order the things that are wanting"

79 John Calvin, *1 & 2 Timothy & Titus: The Crossway Classic Commentaries*, Wheaton, Illinois, 1998, p. 180

80 Acts 27:7-13

81 CS Lewis, *Prince Caspian*, Harper Collins, 1994, p. 184

82 CS Lewis, *Prince Caspian*, Harper Collins, 1994, p. 184

83 https://www.academia.edu/5622061/Doctoral_Thesis_Project_Strengthening_Marriages_BEC

84 An upcoming book in my new Strengthening Health series will on strengthening the marriages of a new generation of healthy leaders.

85 E. Stanley Jones, *Victorious Living*, (Abingdon Press, New York, NY, 1936), p. 341 "

86 The Right Reverend Dr. Silas Ng: http://bishopsilas2.blogspot.ca/; http://discipler123.blogspot.ca.

87 Gene A Getz, *Saying No When You'd Rather Say Yes: Making Choices Based on Titus*, (Regal Books, Ventura, California, 1978), p. 53

88 *Alcoholics Anonymous, the Big Book, Fourth Edition*, (Alcoholic Anonymous World Services, New York, NY, 2013), p. 64

89 Alcoholics Anonymous, p. 66

90 Angus Konstam, p. 13

91 Ephesians 5:18

92 *Alcoholics Anonymous: the Big Book* (Alcohol Anonymous World Services, New York, NY, Third Edition, 1976), p. 58

93 Robert Hilburn, *Johnny Cash: The Life* (Little, Brown, & Company, New York, NY, 2013), p. 538.

94 Hilburn, p. 23.

95 Johnny Cash with Patrick Cash, GK Hall & Co, *The Autobiography: Cash*, (Thorndike, Maine, USA, 1997), p. inside cover, " Johnny Cash 'is in fact the only musician in history to score a triple crown: being inducted into the Songwriter's, Country Music, and Rock and Roll Halls of Fame."

96 Hilburn, p. 104.

97 Hilburn, p. 20.

98 Cash, p. 246

99 *Cash*, edited by Jason Fine (Crown Publishing, New York, NY, 2004), p. 162.

100 Cash. p. 248

101 Cash, p. 261-262

102 *Johnny Cash: My Mother's Hymn Book*, CD liner, p. 15.

103 Cash, p. 299 "A man who really helped me deal with my faith as a public person in the secular world was Billy Graham. He and I spent a lot of time talking the issues over."

104 Hilburn, p. 506.

105 John Carter Cash , *House of Cash: The Legacies of My Father Johnny Cash* (Insight Editions , San Rafael , CA, 2011), p. 55.

106 *Cash*, edited by Jason Fine, p. 149, p. 153. "Really what I discovered, I guess, is myself. I discovered my own self and what makes me tick musically and what I really like. It was really a great inward journey."

107 Hilburn, p. 629.

108 *Johnny Cash: American III: Solitary Man*, 2000, CD liner

109 GK Chesterton, *What's Wrong with the World?*, 'Authority the Unavoidable', Ignatius Press, 1994 http://www.readbookonline.net/read/19314/55248

110 Les Carter and Frank Minirth, *The Anger Workbook* , (Thomas Nelson, 1992), p. 119 "(With pride) anger is inevitable.", p. 153, p. 156.

111 Michael Griffiths, *Timothy and Titus*, (Baker Books, Grand Rapids, Michigan, 1996), p. 133

112 Griffiths, p. 133

113 1 Corinthinans 8:21

114 Brian Kluth, Maximum Generosity website, http://www.kluth.org

115 Matthew 13:14

116 Luke 12:21; James 5:3 "you have heaped up treasure together for the last days"

117 Matthew 6:21 and Luke 12:34

118 2 Corinthians 4:7

119 2 Cor 9:14

120 E. Stanley Jones, *Victorious Living*, p. 5

121 Malachi 3:10 "Bring the whole tithe into the storehouse, that there may be food in my house. Test me in this," says the LORD Almighty, "and see if I will not throw open the floodgates of heaven and pour out so much blessing that there will not be room enough to store it."

122 C.S. Lewis, *Mere Christianity*, Chapter 11 in Book III (Christian Behaviour)

123 Martin Luther King Jr., http://www.serve.gov/?q=site-page/mlkday

124 Romans 12:21; Ephesians 2:10.

125 The Right Reverend Sandy Millar, March 29th 2006 Alpha Clergy Retreat, Cedarsprings Retreat Centre, Sumas, Washington.

126 Proverbs 8:13 "To fear the LORD is to hate evil; I hate pride and arrogance, evil behavior and perverse speech."

127 Michael Griffiths, p. 162

128 Martin Luther, *Three Treatises, A Treatise on Christian Liberty*, LETTER OF MARTIN LUTHER TO POPE LEO X, Wittenberg; 6th September, 1520. (24) p. 297 http://bit.ly/6tqvoK

129 John Wesley, *Rule of Conduct, Letters of John Wesley*, ed. George Eayrs, p. 423, footnote

130 Eric Metaxas, *Amazing Grace: William Wilberforce and the Heroic Campaign to End Slavery*, (HarperCollins Book, New York, NY, 2007), p. 277.

131 *Book of Common Prayer*, ABC Toronto, 1962, p. 13, 14.

132 *Book of Common Prayer*, 1962, p. 4.

133 The Right Reverend Dr. John Rodgers, *Essential Truths for Christians* (Classical Anglican Press, Blue Bell, PA, 2011), p. 403.

134 Kenneth E Bailey, *Finding The Lost: cultural keys to Luke 15*, Concordia, St Louis, MO, 1992, P.168 In the LXX (Septuagint) the verb hygienia almost without exception translates the Hebrew word shalom (peace). It was a good choice because a part of the meaning of shalom is 'good health'.

135 John Calvin, p. 184

136 Dr JI Packer 'Morning Devotional talk', 10th annual Anglican Mission Winter Conference, Greensboro, North Carolina, Sat Jan 20th 2010

137 ANiC Panel (YP Chung, Venables, JI Packer) with Archdeacon Trevor Walters, Friday April 25th 2008

138 Douglas Milne, *Focus on the Bible 1, 2 Timothy & Titus* , (Christian Focus Publications, Great Britain, 1996), p. 208; John 17:3; Gal 4:9; Phil 3:8ff

139 Dr JI Packer, *Reformed Monasticism: History and Theology of the Puritans*, Reformed Theological Seminary, 1988, Reformed Theological Seminary audio talk

140 Hugh Martin, *Puritanism and Richard Baxter*, 1954, SCM Press, London, p. 55: "On Sunday August 17th 1662, some 2,000 ministers took farewell of their parishes, often in the presence of overflowing and weeping congregations. One in five of the clergy were ejected."; Martin, p. 125, "Richard Baxter is usually credited with 168 books"

141 Richard Baxter, *The Saints' Everlasting Rest*, 1652, p. 153 http://www.ccel.org/ccel/baxter/saints_rest.html

142 Dr JI Packer, *Morning Devotions talk*, AMiA Winter Conference 2010, Greensboro, North Carolina

143 Hugh Martin, p. 176; p. 180 "Richard Boyce the scientist said that Richard Baxter feared no man's displeasure, nor hoped for any man's preferment."

144 Hugh Martin, P. 125 "Baxter's influence of the 'Clapham Sect' is just one part of the story of his speaking after death."; p. 131 "(Baxter's) 'Reformed Pastor' influenced Spener, the founder of German Pietism.; p. 146 "Spurgeon (was a) close student of the Puritan preachers, including Baxter."; JI Packer, *A Quest for Godliness: The Puritan Vision of the Christian Life,* Publisher: Crossway Books, 1994

145 http://open.biola.edu/resources/past-watchful-dragons-learning-spiritual-formation-from-c-s-lewis

146 "Dr Jean Houston & the Labyrinth Fad", By Rev Ed Hird, Anglicans for Renewal Canada magazine, May 2,000 http://www3.telus.net/st_simons/armo8.htm

147 Barry Unsworth, *Crete*, National Geographic Society, Washington, DC, 2004 p. 48 In Chania, Crete, is found "the Ikarus Street, named for was the son of the great artificer Daedalus, who built the labyrinth. Father and son were kept imprisoned in this same labyrinth by King Minos. Daedalus made wings for them both out of wax and feathers (but the son flew too close to the sun and the wax melted)."

148 Heritage Walks in Athens, Municipality of Athens Cultural Organization, Athens, Greece, p. 8

149 Hans George Wunderlich, *The Secret of Crete*, (Macmillan Publishing Co, Inc., New York, NY, 1974), p. 44

150 Unsworth, p. 116.

151 During the Nazi takeover of Greece (1936-1941), the Greek Fascist Youth EON (Ethniki Organosi Neolaias) adopted the labyrs as their main symbol. Black Metal fans in Greece still use the labrys as a symbol of Greek Neopaganism. http://en.wikipedia.org/wiki/Labrys (Accessed Nov 26th 2013)

152 Nicholas Platon, Crete, Frederick Muller Limited, London, Nagel Publishers, 1966, p. 183 "...the important part played by the worship of the bull, suggests that the bull symbolized the male creative force and that the bull was worshipped in this form." Some scholars say that the bull was a symbol of Zeus.

153   One Grace Cathedral Labyrinth advocate said that "Labyrinths predate Christianity by over a millennium. The most famous labyrinth from ancient times was the Cretan one, the supposed lair of the mythological Minotaur, which Theseus slew with the aid of Ariadne and her spool of thread rituals…" Peter Corbett, "Pathfinders: Walking medieval labyrinths in a modern world," , p. 2 www.gracecathedral.org/enrichment/features/fea_19981120_txt.shtml (accessed April 1ˢᵗ 2,000); Jean Houston, *Life Force: The Psycho-Historical Recovery of the Self* (Delacorte Press, a division of the Theosophical Publishing House, New York, 1980), p. 263-64 "Now looking at the labyrinth on the floor of Chartres, we remember the searching language of physicists who…describe the structure of our universe as a vortex ring."

154   My 'Yoga: More than Meets the Eyes' article has already been read by more than 75,000 people since April 2013. http://tiny.cc/wg856w

155   Lee Penn, Fall 1999 issue of the Journal of the Spiritual Counterfeits Project www.scp-inc.org http://fatima.freehosting.net/Articles/Art7.htm

156   The Chartres labyrinth dates from sometime between 1194 and 1220. These dates are determined by the great fire of 1194, which destroyed most of the cathedral and the city of Chartres. By 1220 the section of the nave housing the labyrinth had been rebuilt by Bishop Fulbert. Lee Penn LeePenn@aol.com has done careful research showing that the Labyrinth-based relationship between Chartres Cathedral to Grace Cathedral, San Francisco is a clear example of 'the tail wagging the dog', of 'life imitating art'. Grace Cathedral have been giving strong leadership in Chartres' 'reintroduction' of the Labyrinth, even to the point of making Chartres' Dean Legaux an honorary Grace Cathedral Canon.

157   Voices of a New Age Video (1999), Penny Price Productions, E! Online Fact Sheet, "Ten different New Age luminaries voice their view about the possibilities of the human spirit for healing the body, the mind, and the earth."; http://www.eonline.com/Facts/Movies/0,60,53125,00.html (Accessed April 1ˢᵗ 2,000)

158   Jean Houston, GodSeed: the Journey of Christ, Quest Books, The Theosophical Publishing House, Wheaton, USA, 1992, pp. 50, 51. " http://www.jeanhouston.org/store/books/godseed.html (Accessed April 1st 2,000)

159   Robert Todd Carroll, www.skepdic.com/houston.html (accessed May 1998)

160   Bob Woodward in 'The Choice'; The Providence Journal Bulletin, Tuesday, 6/25/96, P. A3

161   www.jeanhouston.org (accessed April 1ˢᵗ 2,000) "drom-e-non. - n. Ancient Gk: a ritual pattern of dynamic expression, a therapeutic dance rhythm in which participants experience second birth into a higher order of consciousness and community;…"

162   www.jeanhouston.org/programs/ms.physical2000/6mstime.html (accessed April 1ˢᵗ 2,000); Houston, *Life Force*, "In 1975, I founded the Dromenon Center, which was named after ancient Greek rites of growth and transformation, in Pomona New York." http://tiny.cc/2tr3fx (accessed May 18ᵗʰ 2014)

163   Jean Houston, *The Possible Human*, Torcher: Houghton, Mifflin Company, 1982, p. ix; Jean Houston, *The Mythic Life*, Harper San Francisco, 1996, p. 186; "Mystery School 1997", http://www.motley-focus.com/mysteryschool97.html (accessed May 18th 2014)

164   www.cathedral.org/cathedral/nca/spiritualperspectives/sacred.html (National Episcopal Cathedral Website) (accessed April 1ˢᵗ 2000) "Keynote speaker, the Reverend Dr. Lauren Artress, Canon for Special Ministries at San Francisco's Grace Cathedral, first encountered a labyrinth in a workshop at psychologist Jean Houston's Mystery School."

165   Houston, *Life Force*, pp. xxv, xviii, xix. http://tiny.cc/2tr3fx (accessed May 18th 2014), "The psycho-technology that Heard advised as providing an initiation of movement from one stage of life to the next was sometimes outrageous and often surreal (LSD, electrical stimulation, walking on fire.)"; http://www.geraldheard.com ; Note: Houston herself was a pioneering LSD researcher 'working with hundreds of research subjects since 1965'.

166   Houston, *Life Force*, p. xxv. http://tiny.cc/2tr3fx (accessed May 18th 2014)

167   H.F. Heard, *The Great Fog: Weird Tales of Terror and Detection* (Vanguard Press, New York, NY, 1944); Houston, *Life Force*, p. 279. http://tiny.cc/2tr3fx (accessed May 18th 2014)

168 Houston, *Life Force*, quoting Heard "Waiting for the Third Act", *London Times Literary Supplement*, June 6th 1960, p. 355ff. "Beyond tragedy lies metacomedy. The central figure of that comedy is known in Asiatic drama… The central figure who dances out of the cosmos, Shiva, consummates laughter and tears in an ecstasis that goes beyond pleasure and pain."; Note: The definitive symbol of yoga is the Nataraj asana, known as the dancing Shiva who 'dances' destruction upon any distinctions (avidya) between the Creator and creation, good and evil, male and female. http://www.theyogatutor.com/natarajasana *The Yoga Teacher*, *Tirusula Yoga*, "Nata= Dancer. Raja = King / Lord" http://bit.ly/TNFTRV (Accessed Dec 23rd 2013).

169 Kristen Fairchild, "A Passion for the Possible: An Interview with Jean Houston," The Spire, Textures 11/04/97 www.gracecathedral.org/enrichment, p. 4, "Jean Houston, Ph.D. is the best-selling author of many books…She has been mentor and teacher of Dr. Lauren Artress, Founder of Veriditas, at Grace Cathedral." (Accessed May 1998)

170 Lauren Artress, *Walking a Sacred Path* (Penguin Group, New York, NY, 1995) p. 2.

171 "Collective Wisdom Initiative: Self-Portrait", Reverend Lauren Artress "The work of symbolic fields has a Jungian base, since I am working with archetypes, symbol, shadow and encounters with collective unconscious." http://www.collectivewisdominitiative.org/files_people/Artress_Lauren.htm (accessed May 18th 2014) Note: Is Artress' Jungian connection merely coincidental or foundational to the Labyrinth fad?

172 Houston, *The Possible Human*, 1982, p. 51

173 Peter Corbett, "Pathfinders: Walking medieval labyrinths in a modern world," http://www.gracecathedral.org/enrichment/features/fea_19981120_txt.shtml "True meditation occurs when the physical brain has been pacified, kept busy with a mantra or a mandala, so the spiritual mind is then free to wander on its own, and discover new truths." states Squires. "…You slowly walk along and slowly walk back, then slowly walk on again." (accessed April 1st 2,000)

174 Occult, according to the Concise Oxford Dictionary, means 'kept secret, esoteric…from the Latin culere: hide' It is not a synonym for Satanism; "…the labyrinth, a sacred tool that has been used as a mandala in many spiritual traditions for thousands of years…" Spiritual Perspectives Program 1996 Sacred Circles Conference http://www.cathedral.org/cathedral/nca/spiritual- perspectives/sacred.html; "The labyrinth is a mandala that meets our longing…" Labyrinth Project, "What Is A Labyrinth," http://www.gracecom.org/veriditas/press/whatlab.shtml, 1996 (accessed April 1st 2,000); http://www3.telus.net/st_simons/arm03.htm "Jung was also a strong promoter of the mandala, a circular picture with a sun or star usually at the centre. Sun worship, as personified in the mandala, is perhaps the key to fully understanding Jung." (ft.103)

175 Houston, *Life Force*, p. 244 "The knower, the knowledge, and the known become part of an undifferentiated unity that is the *unus mundus*, the eternal dance between the One and the Many, the Dromenon."; p. 264 "But in the Dromenon the boundaries between body and soul, other and earth, are effaced." http://tiny.cc/2tr3fx (accessed May 18th 2014); For more on this, you can read my online article "Carl Jung and the Gnostic Reconciliation of Gender Opposites" http://tiny.cc/5uy3fx.

176 http://www.gracecathedral.org/enrichment (accessed April 1st 2,000)

177 www.sfgate.com (accessed April 1st 2,000) Starhawk, as a Wiccan/Witch leader of two covens, celebrated New Year 2,000 by walking the Labyrinth on her San Francisco area Ranch.

178 Lauren Artress, *Walking a Sacred Path: Rediscovering the Labyrinth as a Sacred Tool*, (Riverhead Books/G. P. Putnam's Sons, 1995); sentence quoted by Pamela Sullivan, "Book Review," Pacific Church News, June/July 1995, p. 8

179 Lauren Artress, "Q and A with Lauren," Veriditas, Vol. 1, no. 2, Summer 1996, p. 18

180 www.skepdic.com/houston.html (accessed Nov. 27th 2013)

181 Jean Houston, *The Hero & the Goddess*, (Aquarian/Thorsons , Harper Collins Publisher, 1992), p. 134

182 Dr Jeffrey Satinover, *The Empty Self*, p. 9; Philip Davis,"The Swiss Maharishi", (Touchstone Issue 92, Spring 1996), p.13

183 Nicholas Platon, p. 182

184 Ed Hird, *Battle for the Soul of Canada*, 2006, p. 44, "It is not by accident that virtually every new-age fad, including the DaVinci Code deception, sooner or later draws people into mother/father god/dess worship and sexual immorality. For those wishing to study further on the mother/father god/dess issue, I commend *Speaking the Christian God*, edited by Alvin F. Kimel, Dr. Donald Bloesch *The Battle for the Trinity* and John W Miller's *Biblical Faith and Fathering: why we call God 'Father'*. http://www.anglicanessentials.ca/pdf/montreal_declaration_aec.pdf

185 Douglas Botting, *The Seafarers: The Pirates*, (Time-Life Books Inc., 1978), p. 44 "Whatever the weather, a wooden ship leaked; its planks could seldom be caulked so thoroughly that they let no water in."

186 Douglas Botting, p. 44. "Refuse collected in the bottom of the hull and became a breeding ground for beetles, cockroaches and rats by the scurrying hordes."

187 One of my books in the Strengthening Health series will be a devotional Commentary on 1 Corinthians: strengthening the new generation of healthy small group leaders.

188 E. Stanley Jones, *Victorious Living*, (Abingdon Press, 1936), p. 303

189 Jones, *Victorious Living*, p. 304

190 William Hendriksen, *Commentary on 1st & 2nd Timothy and Titus*, (The Banner of Truth Trust, 1959), p. 352 "These seven (wise men) were : Bias of Priene, Chilon of Sparta, Cleobulus of Lindus, Pittacus of Mitylene, Solon of Athens, Thales of Miletus, and Epimenedes of Crete or Peiander of Corinth or Anacharsis the Scythian."

191 William Barclay, *The Daily Study Bible: The Letters to Timothy, Titus and Philemon*, (GR Welch Co. Ltd., Burlington, Ontario. 1956, 1975), p. 242

192 William Barclay, The Daily Study Bible: The Letters to Timothy, Titus and Philemon, GR Welch Co. Ltd., Burlington, Ontario. 1956, 1975, p. 242

193 George Orwell 1984, http://www.george-orwell.org/1984

194 William Barclay, p. 243 Some commentators compare this to the use of Corinthian as a verb 'to corinthianize' which means to be immoral.

195 William Hendriksen, *Commentary on 1st & 2nd Timothy and Titus*, The Banner of Truth Trust, 1959, p. 354, Cicero, Republic III, ix. 15, 106-43 BC, "Indeed (men's) moral principles are so divergent that the Cretans…consider highway-robbery (or brigandage) to be honorable."

196 Raymond F. Collins, *1 & 2 Timothy and Titus*, (Westminster John Knox Press, Louisville, Kentucky, 2002), p. 137

197 Benjamin Franklin, *Poor Man's Almanac, 1741*

198 C.S. Lewis, *Mere Christianity*, (1952; Harper Collins: 2001), p.198.

199 E Stanley Jones, *Victorious Living*, P. 201

200 Jones, *Victorious Living*, P. 210

201 Thomas Lea and Hayne P. Griffin Jr, *The New American Commentary, 1 & 2 Timothy & Titus*, (Broadman Press, Nashville, Tennessee, 1992), p. 298

202 Dr Gil Stieglitz, ACiC Coaching, Friday May 27th 2005 :

203 Michael Griffiths, *Timothy and Titus*, (Baker Books, Grand Rapids, Michigan, 1996), p. 143.

204 Vancouver Sun, October 2nd 2006, by Bruce Ward, p. A7.

205 Dr Richard Campbell, Semiahmoo, Washington State.

206 Lyle Schaller, *The New Context for Ministry*, (Abingdon Press, Nashville, Tennessee, 2002) p. 13

207 Stuart Briscoe, *Purifying the Church: What God Expects of You and Your Church: A Topical Commentary on Titus*, (Regal Books, GL Publications, 1987), p. 111.

208 Dr Chuck Swindoll, http://john8322.blogspot.com/2010/03/staying-young.html

209 Schlingensiepen, *Dietrich Bonhoeffer: 1906-1945: martyr, thinker, man of resistance*, (T&T Clark, 2010), P.xxii

210 *Valkyrie's Forgotten Man: Dietrich Bonhoeffer*, March 20th 2009, http://bit.ly/dMqnb8

211 Schlingensiepen, P. 10, 228, 382 "chapter 1 ft 6 "the Moravian Losungn (watchword for the day), the daily devotions book, played an operant part in Bonhoeffer's life and is still widely used today."

212 Eric Metaxas, *Bonhoeffer: Pastor, Martyr, Prophet, Spy* , Thomas Nelson,Nashville, P.108

213 *Valkyrie's Forgotten Man: Dietrich Bonhoeffer*, March 20th 2009, http://bit.ly/dMqnb8

214 *Valkyrie's Forgotten Man: Dietrich Bonhoeffer*, http://bit.ly/dMqnb8

215 Metaxas, P.193, P.290 Himmler told Moni Von Cramin: "As an Aryan I must have the courage to take responsibility for my sins alone." He rejected as 'jewish' the idea of putting one's sins on someone else's shoulders.

216 Schlingensiepen, P. 193.

217 Schlingensiepen, P. 205.

218 *Valkyrie's Forgotten Man: Dietrich Bonhoeffer*, http://bit.ly/dMqnb8

219 *Valkyrie's Forgotten Man: Dietrich Bonhoeffer*, http://bit.ly/dMqnb8

220 *Valkyrie's Forgotten Man: Dietrich Bonhoeffer*, http://bit.ly/dMqnb8

221 *Valkyrie's Forgotten Man: Dietrich Bonhoeffer*, http://bit.ly/dMqnb8

222 Schlingensiepen, P. 359.

223 Schlingensiepen, P. 369.

224 Metaxas, P. 464.

225 Michael Griffiths, p. 147.

226 J. Vernon McGee, *Through the Bible, Vol. 5, 1 Corinthians- Revelation*, (Through The Bible Radio, Pasadena, California, 1983), p. 490

227 Thomas Lea and Hayne P. Griffin Jr, *The New American Commentary, 1 & 2 Timothy & Titus*, (Broadman Press, Nashville, Tennessee, 1992), p. 305

228 John Calvin, p. 195.

229 Pascal, *Pensees*, p. 12. http://www.gutenberg.org/files/18269/18269-h/18269-h.htm

230 E Stanley Jones, *Victorious Living*, p. 16.

231 AT Hanson, *The New Century Bible Commentary: The Pastoral Epistles*, (Eerdmans Publishing Company, Grand Rapids, Michigan, 1982), 2:13, p. 186.

232 The Qur'an states that an angel appeared to Mary, to announce to her the "gift of a holy son" (19:19). She was astonished at the news, and asked: "How shall I have a son, seeing that no man has touched me, and I am not unchaste?" (19:20).; the Quran rejects the Deity of Jesus (4:171; 5:17, 70-75; 9:30).

233 E. Stanley Jones, *Victorious Living*, p. 345.

234 Douglas Milne, *Focus on the Bible: 1, 2 Timothy & Titus*, (Christian Focus Publications, Great Britain, 1996), p. 11 " The theological stance of the Pastorals is 'epiphanic', meaning by this that its teachings and appeals are firmly framed within the two great epiphanies or appearings of Jesus Christ. (1 Tim. 3:16;6:14;2 Tim 1:10; 4:1, 8; Titus 2:11, 13; 3:4)."

235 Al-Imran 3:52-55; An-Nissa 4:156-159.

236 *Book of Common Prayer, The Communion*, p. 82.

237 An upcoming book in my Strengthening Health series is Emotional Cutoff: strengthening the new generation of healthy leaders through family wisdom.

238 Sam Shoemaker, *If I be Lifted Up*, (New York: Fleming H. Revell, Ada, Michigan, 1931), p. 26-27,

239 Henry Blackaby, 'EXPERIENCING God Together: For Such a Time as This' Conference with *More Than Gold*, Fraserview Church, Richmond, March 7th 2009

240 William Barclay, *The Daily Study Bible: The Letters to Timothy, Titus and Philemon*, (GR Welch Co. Ltd., Burlington, Ontario. 1956, 1975), p. 258

241 John Calvin, *1 & 2 Timothy & Titus*

242 John Stott, *Guard the Truth: The Message of 1 Timothy & Titus*, (Inter-Varsity Press, Downers Grove, Illinois, 1996).

243 John Calvin, p. 205.

244 An upcoming book in my Strengthening Health series will be on Incarnational Renewal: strengthening the new generation of healthy renewal leaders.

245 John Calvin, p. 207.

246 Walter Isaacson, *Benjamin Franklin: An American Life*, (Simon and Schuster, New York, 2003), , p. 317

247 "Benjamin Franklin's Private Fleet", National Geographic Channel, http://natgeotv.com/asia/ben-franklins-pirate-fleet. (accessed Dec. 23rd 2013)

248 "Privateering, the American Revolution, and the Rules of War", History News Network, http://hnn.us/article/915.; John Frayler "Privateers in the American Revolution", Salem Maritime National Historic Site http://www.nps.gov/revwar/about_the_revolution/privateers.html (accessed Dec 23rd 2013)

249 Isaacson, p. 99.

250 Isaacson, p. 468

251 Isaacson, p. 482.

252 Benjamin Franklin, *Poor Richard's Almanac*, (Peter Pauper Press, Inc, White Plains, NY,1952), p. v.; Isaacson, p. 264.

253 Isaacson, p. 264, p. 426.

254 Isaacson, p. 265.

255 Isaacson, p. 182, p. 257, p. 479.

256 Isaacson, p. 257, p. 303.

257 Isaacson, p. 312 "He (BF) crossed out, using the heavy backslashes that he often employed, the last three words of Jefferson's phrase: 'We hold these truths to be sacred and undeniable' and changed them to the words now enshrined in history: 'We hold these truths to be self-evident.'

258 Isaacson, p. 316, p. 459.

259 Isaacson, p. 327, p. 347-8.

260 William P. Grady, *What Hath God Wrought!*, pp.104-105.

261 Benjamin Franklin letter dated March 1778 to the Ministry of France.

262 Benjamin Franklin, "Speech to the Constitutional Convention", 1787, http://www.pioneernet.net/rbrannan/whitefield/bfongw.htm ; Isaacson, p. 467.

263 Isaacson, pp. 463-464.; http://www.archives.gov/legislative/features/franklin/ ; http://tiny.cc/fknn8w (accessed Dec 25th 2013)

264 Franklin, *Poor Richard's Almanac*, p. 77.

CPSIA information can be obtained at www.ICGtesting.com
Printed in the USA
LVOW08s0709170914

404369LV00006B/17/P